COSMETIC
LASER
SURGERY

COSMETIC

LASER

SURGERY

———

Edited by

Tina S. Alster, M.D.

Director, Washington Institute of Dermatologic Laser Surgery
Assistant Clinical Professor of Dermatology and Pediatrics
Georgetown University Medical Center
Washington, D.C.

David B. Apfelberg, M.D.

Director, Atherton Plastic Surgery Center
Atherton, California
Assistant Clinical Professor of Plastic Surgery
Stanford University Medical Center

ⓦ WILEY-LISS

A JOHN WILEY & SONS, INC., PUBLICATION
New York • Chichester • Brisbane • Toronto • Singapore

While the authors, editor, and publisher believe that drug selection and dosage and the specification and usage of equipment and devices, as set forth in this book, are in accord with current recommendations and practice at the time of publication, they accept no legal responsibility for any errors or omissions, and make no warranty, express or implied, with respect to material contained herein. In view of ongoing research, equipment modifications, changes in governmental regulations and the constant flow of information relating to drug therapy, drug reactions, and the use of equipment and devices, the reader is urged to review and evaluate the information provided in the package insert or instructions for each drug, piece of equipment, or device for, among other things, any changes in the instructions or indication of dosage or usage and for added warnings and precautions.

Library of Congress Cataloging in Publication Data:

Cosmetic laser surgery / editors, Tina S. Alster, David B. Apfelberg.
      p. cm.
      Includes bibliographical references and index.
      ISBN 0-471-12242-4 (cloth : alk. paper)
      1. Surgery, Plastic.   2. Lasers in Surgery.   I. Alster, Tina S.
II. Apfelberg, David B.
      [DNLM: 1. Surgery, Plastic.   2. Laser Surgery.   WO 600 C8335
1996]
      RD119.C65   1996
      617.9'5—dc20
      DNLM/DLC
      for Library of Congress   95–25054
                                           CIP

Printed in the United States of America

10 9 8 7 6 5 4 3 2 1

CONTENTS

─────

6 LASER-ASSISTED UVULOPALATOPLASTY FOR SNORING   67

Yosef P. Krespi, M.D. and Maurice M. Khosh, M.D.

7 LASER TREATMENT OF SCARS   81

Tina S. Alster, M.D.

8
LASER TREATMENT OF TELANGIECTASIAS   93

Heidi A. Waldorf, M.D., Gary P. Lask, M.D., and Roy G. Geronemus, M.D.

9
LASER TREATMENT OF TATTOOS AND PIGMENTED LESIONS   111

Suzanne L. Kilmer, M.D. and Tina S. Alster, M.D.

CONTRIBUTORS

Tina S. Alster, M.D.
Director, Washington Institute of Dermatologic Laser Surgery
Assistant Clinical Professor of Dermatology and Pediatrics
Georgetown University Medical Center
Washington, D.C.

David B. Apfelberg, M.D.
Director, Atherton Plastic Surgery Center
Atherton, California
Assistant Clinical Professor of Plastic Surgery
Stanford University Medical Center
Stanford, California

Roy G. Geronemus, M.D.
Director, Laser and Skin Surgery Center of New York
New York University Medical Center
New York, New York

Gregory S. Keller, M.D.
Director, Keller Facial Plastic Surgery Clinic and Laser Center
Santa Barbara, California
Assistant Professor, UCLA Medical Center

Maurice M. Khosh, M.D.
Roosevelt Hospital
New York, New York

Suzanne L. Kilmer, M.D.
Director, Laser and Skin Surgery Center of Northern California
Sacramento, California
University of California–Davis School of Medicine

Yosef P. Krespi, M.D.
Director, Department of Otolaryngology
Roosevelt Hospital
Professor, College of Physicians and Surgeons
Columbia University
New York, New York

Gary P. Lask, M.D.
Director, Dermatology Laser Center
UCLA School of Medicine
Director of Dermatologic Surgery and Research
Harbor–UCLA Medical Center
Torrance, California

Walter P. Unger, M.D.
Hospital of the University of Toronto
Toronto, Ontario, Canada

Heidi A. Waldorf, M.D.
Fellow, Laser and Skin Surgery Center of New York
New York, New York

Cynthia Weinstein, M.D.
Department of Plastic Surgery
Freemasons Hospital-Day Procedure Center
East Melbourne, Australia

FOREWORD

The very first medical use of lasers was for skin lesions by Dr. Leon Goldman. More than 30 years later, lasers have become widely accepted for treatment of microvascular malformations, pigmented lesions, tattoos, controlled vaporization, and coagulation. A dozen different lasers are now produced for dermatology, many of which are designed for specific uses.

Progress in laser surgery comes from a combination of new technology, basic science, clinical exploration, and serendipitous discovery. The matrix of lasers and their applications is constantly expanding, which is confusing to anyone starting to use these remarkable tools. In particular, we have learned that "targeting" of laser light absorption and heating of specific skin structures brings a level of specificity and surgical control unique to lasers. My fascination with lasers began and continues this way, so I have to remind myself and many of my patients that lasers really aren't magic bullets. The tissue selectivity, precision, and hemostasis of lasers make them useful tools. Like all surgical tools, they can also be grossly destructive and dangerous when misused. Goldman's classic advice, "If you don't need a laser, don't use one" is well worth repeating here. This book helps us better define the need for particular lasers in cosmetic surgery.

The skin is a resilient organ, adapted for direct contact with a harsh environment. In some ways, this is a book about what we can do to skin *without* inducing a scar. And, it is rather amazing. When we use a pulsed dye laser to selectively destroy most of the circulatory system in the upper 1-2 mm, a process begins of local remodeling and replacement neovascularization, without scarring. This is great for treatment of telangiectasia. Remarkably, Dr. Alster recently found that pulsed dye laser treatment benefits existing scars, remodeling the surface texture closer to that of normal skin. When we use short laser pulses absorbed by melanin, most or all of the epidermal melanocytes and pigmented keratinocytes are destroyed, then replaced. When we pulse or scan a CO_2 laser for "resurfacing" the entire epidermis and upper dermis is vaporized, followed by repair that leaves an improved cosmetic appearance. The better surgical precision and hemostasis make laser resurfacing attractive compared with chemical peels or dermabrasion.

Pictures really are worth thousands of words, especially when aesthetics are the topic. With this picture-filled book, Tina Alster and David Apfelberg offer us a needed, user-friendly atlas and guide to cosmetic laser surgery. Enjoy.

R. ROX ANDERSON, M.D.

PREFACE

Since their first development more than three decades ago, lasers have assumed an increasingly important role in the treatment of cutaneous lesions. Beginning with the pioneering work of Dr. Leon Goldman in the 1960s with the ruby laser, a proliferation of reports using a variety of laser systems to treat a myriad of dermatologic conditions ensued. As technology advanced, newer lasers were developed which took advantage of the unique characteristics of absorption by specific targets (or chromophores) in the skin using high energy, short pulses that limited unnecessary thermal injury. This theoretical concept of "selective photothermolysis" proposed by Drs. Rox Anderson and John Parrish in the early 1980s paved the way for the development of lasers specifically designed to remove pigmented, vascular, and tattooed cutaneous lesions.

As experience accumulated demonstrating the benefits of lasers for excision, ablation, and reconstruction, it became apparent that the same technology could be applied in the cosmetic arena. Further refinement of laser technology, such as "ultra"-pulsing of the carbon dioxide laser, Q-switching of the ruby, alexandrite, and Nd:YAG lasers, and developing sapphire tips and sculpted fibers for the Nd:YAG laser, has contributed to these advances. As a result, ablation or excision can now be accomplished in a relatively bloodless manner, utilizing lasers with "cold" beams that eliminate the potential of thermal or burn tissue injury. Reports have indicated substantially reduced bleeding, bruising, swelling, and pain following these laser-assisted procedures. Thus, innovative surgeons have applied new laser principles to such common and traditional procedures as skin resurfacing, tattoo removal, scar revision, hair transplantation, and facial cosmetic surgery with markedly improved results.

There is no doubt with the reforms proposed in several health-care systems throughout the world, that the use of lasers in outpatient settings will outdistance their use in operating rooms. In fact, office-based laser procedures in dermatology, plastic surgery, ophthalmology, and otolaryngology are leading the way in the medical-laser industry. Through this book, we have attempted to summarize the current utilization of multiple lasers for a variety of cosmetic procedures. Leading laser specialists from a variety of fields have contributed their experiences, treatment protocols, and assessments on the use of lasers for everything from skin resurfacing to uvula-palatoplasty. Clinical cases in each chapter have been highlighted with appropriate laser parameters and treatment guidelines in order to assist the reader in selecting the proper treatment protocol for some of the most common cosmetic conditions encountered. A detailed appendix with sample consent forms, operative reports, office treatment charting forms, and referral letters will help organize practitioners new to these laser procedures.

Undoubtedly, further clinical experience and research will offer additional insights and promote technique modifications using these and other laser systems. We feel privileged to be able to offer laser surgery as a viable treatment option to our patients and to be part of an ever-growing team of physicians and scientists interested in expanding our knowledge of lasers in medicine and surgery.

Washington, D.C.   TINA S. ALSTER, M.D.
Atherton, California   DAVID B. APFELBERG, M.D.

ACKNOWLEDGMENTS

We extend our gratitude to all those who have contributed directly and indirectly in the preparation of this book. Each author is considered to be an expert in his or her own discipline and, thus, we feel fortunate that we were given an opportunity to include their individual approaches and innovative procedures. The fact that the book was conceived of and developed in such a short time makes each contribution that much more valuable and appreciated.

We acknowledge, as well, the patient and creative efforts of our colleagues and staff who tolerated our fits of frenzy, as last minute requests and "lost" data searches were made.

Our deepest appreciation goes to our spouses, Paul Frazer and Susan Apfelberg, without whose understanding, support, and encouragement we could not have completed this project.

To our editor, Shawn Morton, who had the vision to recognize the potential contribution of this book in furthering medical education and patient treatment.

Finally, a special thanks to our patients who allow us to draw from their personal experiences in order to expand our clinical knowledge and develop further treatments.

T.S.A.
D.B.A.

COSMETIC
LASER
SURGERY

1

EVALUATION, INSTALLATION, AND MARKETING OF A COSMETIC LASER PRACTICE

Tina S. Alster, M.D.

David B. Apfelberg, M.D.

1.1 INTRODUCTION

The decision to add a laser to a practice, emphasizing primarily cosmetic surgery, requires careful study. Basically, the choice of laser systems includes the following technologies: Q-switched lasers for tattoos and pigmented lesions; pulsed (or tunable) dye lasers for vascular, pigmented, and scarred lesions; high-energy pulsed carbon dioxide lasers for hair transplantation, uvula palatoplasty to alleviate snoring, and skin resurfacing of rhytides and atrophic scars; and Nd:YAG or carbon dioxide lasers for facial cosmetic surgeries, such as meloplasty and blepharoplasty.

Because lasers are expensive to obtain and maintain, careful consideration must be given to many factors, including economic realities, community needs, referral network, marketing strategies, and personal interest, before a final decision should be reached.

1.2 EVALUATION OF YOUR PRACTICE

A careful review of one's patient mix or practice profile is the first step in determining whether the addition of a laser is appropriate (Table 1.1). Is the practice primarily medical, reconstructive, or cos-

Cosmetic Laser Surgery, Edited by Alster, M.D. and Apfelberg, M.D.
ISBN 0471-12242-4 © 1996 Wiley-Liss, Inc.

2

TABLE 1.1   Laser Practice Checklist

- **What is your practice profile?**
  - **Medical versus reconstructive versus cosmetic**
  - **Pediatric versus adult versus geriatric**
  - **Referral network**
  - **Private pay versus insurance versus Medicare**
- **Do you have adequate training?**
- **Is there room for a laser?**
- **Is your staff prepared?**
- **Are you aware of applicable laser safety and malpractice issues?**
- **What is the local market?**
- **Is there existing competition?**
- **Can you really afford a laser?**

metic? Practices of a more cosmetic bend will naturally be more amenable to the addition of a laser. Is the patient population young or old? With the exception of children with vascular and pigmented birthmarks, most laser surgeries are performed on older individuals with years of chronic sun exposure and subsequent development of lentigines, rhytides, and telangiectasias. Are patients presenting with problems that could better be treated with lasers or are they already requesting alternative forms of treatment? For instance, patients who have received unsuccessful treatment with cryosurgery for lentigines or electrosurgery for rosacea may demand more selective laser treatment. Do patients with tattoos and scars commonly present for treatment? Prior to the use of the most recent lasers, treatment of these conditions was limited due to excessive scarring or pigmentary alteration.

While it is true that older patients have more lesions that are amenable to laser treatment, those who are eligible for Medicare may not avail themselves of cosmetic services. Thus the payor mix of one's patient population should be studied. If the majority of patients have managed care plans, for instance, a significant barrier to treatment is encountered, as many plans exclude laser treatment on cosmetic grounds. On the other hand, a certain proportion of the patients who desire treatment may elect to become private-pay patients if they have the extra monetary resources. Certainly, laser treatment of extensive lesions, such as birthmarks and scars, may be approved for reimbursement by many insurance companies on a case-by-case basis.

The referral pattern of one's practice should also be given consideration when contemplating the purchase of a laser. Does the physician enjoy a reputation of excellence with a wide range of referring primary care doctors who would be enthusiastic about a new technology? Or does the practice depend on word-of-mouth referrals from established patients who may not appreciate the "newness" of the laser? Are lasers currently used in the practice so that referring physicians and patients would readily accept the new laser procedure? Or is the laser totally new to the practice, requiring patients, referring doctors, and office staff to learn an entirely new treatment modality? Does the laser enhance skills already learned (e.g., hair transplantation and blepharoplasty), or does it require extensive training in *two* new skills?

1.3 FUTURE PRACTICE DIRECTION

The addition of a laser to a practice could potentially perk up a boring practice. The laser may attract a totally new group of patients or stimulate a new list of referring physicians. A medical or reconstructive insurance-based practice may be converted into a more cosmetic private-pay enterprise. Many physicians find that the laser portion of their practices serves as an enhancer for other cosmetic activities. It is not unusual, for instance, for a patient who presents for treatment of acne rosacea or solar lentigines to inquire about a chemical peel, basic skin care regimen, or even a blepharoplasty or facelift! Since these patients are already focused on cosmetic self-improvement, they are also often interested in ancillary and, many times, more extensive and expensive procedures.

1.4 EVALUATION OF EXTERNAL FACTORS

An assessment of the community and existing competition is essential. A very sophisticated area with numerous lasers and medical centers may not justify the addition of another laser, as the general population is already being adequately served. On the other hand, a physician who is first to offer a unique laser service to the community may have a built-in advantage. It is important to remember that the immediately adjacent locales are no longer considered to be the only geographic "draw" areas, as patients will often travel long distances for a perceived unique or better "high-tech" treatment. It is not necessary, however, to be the only laser practice in town. The presence of a competitive laser in one's geographic area may serve to heighten awareness of the community at large to the attributes of lasers so that several practices could sustain ample laser activity. In addition, competing lasers may actually complement each other, so that green tattoos that are less successfully removed by the Nd:YAG laser, for example, could be treated by a competitor's alexandrite or ruby laser. Laser physicians could potentially work with each other to the benefit of all involved.

4

1.5 EVALUATION OF YOUR OFFICE AND PERSONNEL

Several aspects of one's office and staff should be taken into consideration prior to committing to a laser purchase. For instance, does a particular room already exist that can accommodate a laser and its accessories or does one need to be specifically built for that purpose? While most lasers do not require special electrical wiring, some may need water cooling. In addition, excessive heat may be produced in small rooms, so adequate ventilation should be considered. If windows exist in a treatment room, it will be necessary to cover them with opaque material. Proper placement of anesthetic equipment, lighting, smoke evacuators, and other supplies need to be addressed. The type of safety measures and staff training required will depend on the type of laser installed and prior laser experience of the staff. OSHA or malpractice requirements could potentially be changed with the addition of a laser.

It is absolutely essential that all office staff be well-versed in the clinical applications of the laser. Receptionists, in particular, are commonly faced with potential patients desiring detailed information regarding the laser services offered. Additionally, it is imperative that phone access and scheduling be adequate. It is counterproductive to have interested and excited patients calling the office, only to find that an appointment cannot be scheduled for many weeks. These patients often lose interest if not seen in a reasonable time period or may seek another specialist with similar laser capabilities.

1.6 OBTAINING LASER CERTIFICATION

While there are no specific guidelines for laser certification, it is generally agreed that a basic laser course covering general laser principles and some clinical "hands-on" training are imperative before a physician begins performing laser treatments on his or her own (Table 1.2). Reading the existing laser surgery literature in one's specialty is additionally helpful before attending a laser course so that the terminology is somewhat familiar. The laser field is growing so rapidly that much of what is being discovered is being incorporated immediately into clinical practice before it is ever published.

TABLE 1.2   Using Lasers Like an Expert—Getting Certified

- Obtain initial and ongoing education: read laser articles and books
- Attend laser seminars
- Get "hands-on" training
- Join appropriate laser societies

5

Therefore it is important to not only obtain the initial basic training but to stay abreast of ongoing changes and advances by attending laser seminars at specialty meetings and laser societies.

1.7 CHOOSING THE CORRECT LASER FOR YOU

Various laser manufacturers should be canvassed for a description of their equipment, maintenance plans, and service availability. Obviously, the basic laser price is a major consideration, but other costs that should be considered include service or maintenance contracts and "disposibles," such as dye cartridges. Scrutiny of the installed base of the laser company is important in order to determine its financial strength and future longevity. Many laser companies have a major corporate support that ensures the long-term success of the laser division. Pending FDA approvals for all laser applications should be known.

Make sure to order the latest, most technically advanced laser model available. If major improvements or model changes are contemplated, make certain that an upgrade will be forthcoming at minimal or no cost. The availability of a local laser representative or technician is often very useful in the event of medical or technical problems. Laser installation with a 1-year service contract and appropriate physician and staff training are provided by most companies as part of a laser sale.

1.8 LASER OPTIONS: HOW TO OBTAIN A LASER

Laser costs can be evaluated using strict accounting methods of amortization analysis. The price of the laser, accessories, maintenance, and disposibles is computed and divided by the useful life of the laser (approximately 5 years) to obtain annual costs. These costs are then divided by the number of cases predicted to be performed per year to determine the cost per procedure. Expenses can then be passed directly to the patient or be absorbed into the practice overhead costs in exchange for a larger, revenue-building patient population. (Table 1.3).

TABLE 1.3 To Lease or Buy?—That is the Question

LEASE	BUY
• Less initial investment	• More capital needed
• More flexible upgrade options	• Less flexibility with equipment changes
• Monthly business deductions	• Depreciation deductions over time
• Trade-in at term's end	• It's yours

6

The decision to lease or buy a laser should take into consideration several factors. Leasing allows for improved cash flow, as less capital is invested initially. This may be especially important to new practitioners who do not have the capital to invest in a sizable downpayment. Additionally, many leasing companies offer better finance rates so that payments are lower than when purchasing. Leasing high-technology equipment allows for greater flexibility with regard to upgrades or trade-ins so that one is not encumbered with obsolete equipment at the end of a lease term. Lastly, immediate business deductions can be taken over the life of the lease rather than claiming the depreciation over the useful life of purchased equipment.

Mobile laser units have added another possible option for practitioners who are considering the addition of a laser to their armamentarium of treatments. Essentially, one could arrange for delivery of a particular laser to the office on certain days of the month and schedule all laser patients accordingly. This type of setup allows for the least amount of money invested in equipment with maximal usage. Drawbacks to the mobile laser units include scheduling limitations as other practitioners share laser time, possible increase in laser malfunction due to inherent shifting of laser parts with repeated equipment moves, and decreased income tax advantages. On the other hand, the mobile units allow a practitioner to become familiar with the laser technology and provide time for the laser practice to be established before a final commitment is made to buy or lease.

1.9 MARKETING YOUR LASER PRACTICE

To make the laser purchase worthwhile and successful, a sufficient patient volume must be generated. In addition to one's established patients who wish to avail themselves of the new technology, a whole new generation of patients not previously serviced by the practice will be enticed. There are multiple ways of promoting or marketing one's new laser capability (Table 1.4).

Probably the easiest and least expensive way to promote a laser practice is by word of mouth. Just chatting with established

TABLE 1.4 The Short Course on Marketing

- Word-of-mouth
- Informational letters and brochures to patients and referring physicians
- Special events—health fairs, community outreach programs
- Lectures/announcements—medical societies, grand rounds, service groups, health clubs, beauty salons
- Direct (paid) advertising—newspaper, magazine, TV, radio
- Indirect advertising—PR firm, TV or local newspaper/magazine story
- Publications—medical literature

patients, family, and friends about your "exciting new laser" often pays off in referrals. Prior to actually installing the laser, many office patients or phone shoppers who inquire about laser treatment should be kept on a separate list for recall and mailing. It is amazing how a laser waiting list can grow during the time it takes for you to evaluate its feasibility in your practice.

A short informational letter on your letterhead, accompanied by a simple color graphic or logo, should be sent to prospective patients, referring physicians, and other business contacts. The letter should be personal enough to convey the excitement and ability to provide new laser services, but should also contain information about the types of conditions amenable to laser treatment, general guidelines with respect to the time and cost of treatment, efficacy rate and possible side effects, as well as insurance factors. Letters should also be sent to associated specialists (beyond dermatologists and plastic surgeons) who may have an interest in sending patients for laser treatment: for instance, pediatricians for vascular and pigmented birthmarks, geriatricians for solar lentigines and telangiectasias, and general or thoracic surgeons for scars are all possible sources of referrals.

Descriptive flyers or brochures with "before and after" laser treatment color photographs can be obtained through the laser manufacturer or designed personally by the physician. They should accompany letters and be displayed in the office to attract patient interest. In addition, laser manufacturers often provide a package of marketing and practice enhancement suggestions, including sample letters, brochures, videos, and radio and TV advertisements to aid in the successful establishment of a laser practice.

Special events, such as health fairs and community outreach programs, are excellent avenues at which to promote one's laser practice. In one area, a physician with a new tattoo laser offered to treat, without charge, gang members as part of a rehabilitation and job enhancement program through the local social service agency. This generous offer was widely publicized in the news with personal interviews and resulted in the addition of several private-pay patients to the practice as well.

Lectures at local medical society meetings or hospital grand rounds serve to educate local physicians about laser surgery. House staff and nurses at area hospitals are excellent sources of referrals. In addition, informational seminars for lay groups, such as community service clubs (Rotary, Kiwanis, Elks), church groups, health clubs, and beauty salons, are an excellent way to spread the word about laser surgery. Some physicians even sponsor "open to the public" lectures, given at a hotel, rented hall, or hospital auditorium, which is promoted by notice in the local newspaper, hospital bulletin board or newsletter, and patient mailers. Similarly, "open house" tours of the office or laser facility may be effective in introducing physicians and prospective patients to the technology.

8

Paid advertising in newspapers, in magazines, on radio, and on television is another viable marketing option, although costs can be considerable. If one is fortunate enough to peak the interest of a local journalist to laser surgery, the result could be a free advertisement in the form of a magazine or newspaper article! Writers, producers, and TV personalities, by sheer virtue of their public personae, may best appreciate the benefits of cosmetic laser surgery. Hiring a public relations consultant to "bridge the gap" between the medical aspects of the practice and the promotional aspects can save one time and lead to a more effective marketing campaign, since publicists often have press contacts that are not readily available to most physicians and can more easily relate the facts of the surgery in terms a layperson can understand.

Lastly, delivering presentations to other physicians at national medical and laser surgery meetings on one's laser experience and results of clinical trials not only provides a forum during which vital information is shared and knowledge enhanced by other practitioners, but also can lead to referrals for treatment. While the publication of medical articles can be cumbersome, the dissemination of knowledge and novel techniques adds to the overall education of others about laser surgery and to their perception of you as an excellent laser resource.

SKIN RESURFACING WITH HIGH ENERGY, PULSED CARBON DIOXIDE LASERS

Cynthia Weinstein, M.D.

Tina S. Alster, M.D.

2.1 INTRODUCTION

Since the development of the first laser by Dr. Theodore Maiman in 1960 (1), laser applications in cosmetic surgery have expanded considerably. The early continuous-wave lasers, although producing major advances in the treatment of several cutaneous lesions, were limited by their nonspecific thermal effects. Improvements in laser technology utilizing the theory of selective photothermolysis have enabled the use of pulsed laser systems, which minimize thermal injury to noninvolved tissues (2–4). Nowhere has this been more clearly demonstrated than with the use of hemoglobin-specific pulsed dye lasers, which revolutionized the treatment of vascular lesions, especially port-wine stains (5–9).

Carbon dioxide lasers, emitting light at 10,600 nanometers (nm), have maintained a prominent position in dermatology and cosmetic surgery over the past few decades due to their broad range of applications. In a focused mode, continuous-wave (CW) carbon dioxide lasers can cut through tissues with a marked reduction in bleeding (10), being especially useful for surgeries in highly vascular areas, such as the face and scalp. Laser-assisted blepharoplasties and facelifts have consequently become more popular (11–14). CW carbon dioxide lasers are also used in the defocused mode to vaporize

Cosmetic Laser Surgery, Edited by Alster, M.D. and Apfelberg, M.D.
ISBN 0471-12242-4   © 1996 Wiley-Liss, Inc.

10

tissue, allowing recontouring of skin in cases of rhinophyma (15–17) or removal of photodamaged tissue in actinic cheilitis (18–21). Advantages of carbon dioxide laser surgery over traditional excisional surgery include a reduction in bruising and swelling, quicker patient recovery, and better visualization of tissues during surgery (22,23).

Despite these clear advantages, use of the continuous-wave carbon dioxide laser for skin resurfacing had been limited by excessive heat conduction to normal surrounding skin with resultant scarring and pigmentary changes. Thus, dermabrasion and chemical peels continued to be the preferred treatments for improving the appearance of acne scars and photodamaged skin despite several drawbacks, even in the most experienced hands. With dermabrasion, in particular, bleeding during the procedure made visualization of the actual treatment endpoint difficult. In addition, the relatively large, bulky instruments impeded the sculpting of fine wrinkles and indentations. As such, a significant risk of scarring (especially on the upper lip and philtrum) and hypopigmentation remained. The persistent aerosol produced by dermabrasion also posed a significant risk of viral transmission from patient to patient and from patient to medical personnel (24). The multiple individual and technique-dependent variables contributing to the effectiveness of a chemical peel, including the type and concentration of chemicals used, the preparation of the skin prior to peeling, the method of chemical application, the contact time of the chemical with the skin, and post-treatment care (including taping), similarly limited the standardization of results achieved by chemical treatment (25).

In response to the problems of excessive thermal damage occurring in normal tissue due to heat diffusion from CW carbon dioxide laser-irradiated skin, carbon dioxide lasers have recently been developed that use high peak powers with rapid pulses. The new "ultra-pulsed" capabilities diminish thermal conduction by limiting the pulse duration to shorter than the target tissue thermal relaxation time (26–33). As such, clean ablation of cutaneous lesions can be achieved with minimal damage to normal skin by vaporizing the lesional tissue faster than heat can be conducted to the surrounding area. These high-energy, pulsed carbon dioxide lasers are therefore ideally suited to resurfacing skin abnormalities, creating a "what you see is what you get" effect on human tissue.

Because the rate of ablation depends on the irradiance or power density, a critical irradiance needs to be exceeded for minimal thermal damage to occur. The critical irradiance for carbon dioxide laser surgery on skin surfaces is 200 watts/mm^2 to produce a 0.02-millimeter (mm) zone of minimal thermal damage (34). When ablation is attempted at less than the critical irradiance, overheating with subsequent charring and/or scarring may result. Charring can be avoided by lasing at power densities greater than the critical value.

Thus working at lower irradiances in the interest of safety and precision may produce exactly the opposite result.

The first pulsed carbon dioxide lasers ("superpulsed") produced high spiked peak power followed by a tail of lower power so that the power density actually exceeded the critical value for only a brief time period. Thus the energy delivered was only slightly enhanced over the continuous-wave carbon dioxide lasers. The newer radiofrequency discharge lasers ("ultrapulsed") produce higher peak power but maintain the peak throughout the entire pulse, resulting in significantly greater pulse energy (Figure 2.1). Effective pulsing requires a frequency of less than 1000 pulses per second and a pulse length of less than one-third of the time between pulses. Clean, bloodless, and char-free tissue ablation requires that a single laser impact contain enough energy [minimum of 250 millijoules (mJ) at a 3-mm spot size] to vaporize the lesional tissue so that the remnants can be cleared before heat is conducted to normal adjacent

11

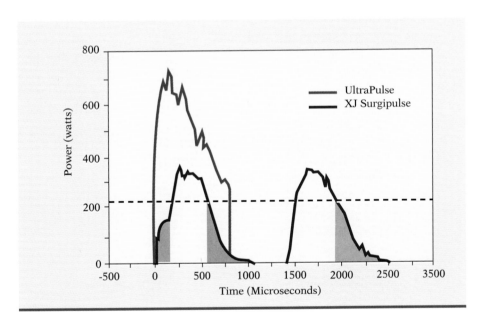

FIGURE 2.1 The *dashed line* represents the threshold power required for minimal residual thermal damage for a 3-mm wide beam from a carbon dioxide laser. Thermal damage is minimal for irradiances above 200 watts/mm^2, which corresponds to 225 watts for a 3-mm beam. The *shaded area* represents times for which greater than minimal thermal damage occurs. The total pulse energy for each laser was set to 400 mJ. The pulse shapes and peak powers were determined with a fast pyroelectric detector. The XJ Surgipulse waveform showed two 200-mJ pulses, whereas the Ultrapulse showed a single high-energy pulse without falling below the 225-watt threshold irradiance.

12

structures. Thus tissue vaporization is maximized and heat buildup in adjacent areas is eliminated through adequate cooling of tissue between pulses.

2.2 INDICATIONS FOR CARBON DIOXIDE LASER RESURFACING PROCEDURE

Shortly after the introduction of the new high-energy, pulsed carbon dioxide laser technology, indications for its use in skin resurfacing increased substantially. While the older continuous-wave and "superpulsed" lasers were useful in resurfacing rhinophyma, actinic cheilitis, and acne scars, the "ultrapulsed" lasers have superseded their predecessors for use in a number of cosmetic situations due to their improved laser–tissue interaction (35–39).

Rhytides caused by excessive ultraviolet exposure are very suitable for carbon dioxide laser resurfacing (Table 2.1). The most commonly encountered rhytides of this type are located periorbitally and periorally, though they can also occur on the cheeks, ears, nose, and chest. The small (3-mm) spot size of the current laser systems make lasing large areas tedious and time-consuming, but recent advances in technology have allowed for even large areas to be resurfaced rapidly. Some physicians prefer to supplement the current laser technology with chemical peels when treating large surface areas. Using this approach, deeper wrinkles are first resurfaced with the laser and then the surrounding areas peeled with a more superficial agent than usual in order to blend in with the remaining cosmetic unit. With the lower concentration of acid, the risk of scarring or pigmentary changes is further minimized.

Rhytides that result from muscle activity, such as those in the glabellar or nasolabial folds, do not respond as favorably to laser

TABLE 2.1 Laser Resurfacing: Indications for Treatment

	INDICATIONS	CONTRAINDICATIONS
Primary	Perioral rhytides Periorbital rhytides Atrophic (pitted) scars Benign cutaneous growths	Oral retinoid use
Secondary	Glabellar rhytides Forehead rhytides Nasolabial folds	Dark (olive) skin tone Ultraviolet light exposure Prior treatment with resultant scarring

resurfacing. It has been noted, however, that frown lines, in particular, can be improved with the laser resurfacing procedure, but that they may recur more readily than those rhytides caused by non-muscular or actinic damage (T.S. Alster, *personal communication*).

Pulsed carbon dioxide laser resurfacing of scars from acne, surgery, and trauma have shown results superior to other forms of treatment. In general, scars that are pitted or atrophic are best suited to laser ablation. Additionally, resurfacing of potentially hypertrophic or keloidal scars at 6–8 weeks following surgery or trauma can attenuate their appearance so that they blend well with surrounding normal skin. It is important to time the procedure to maximize collagen reorganization during the normal wound repair mechanism in order to prevent visible scar tissue from forming.

The carbon dioxide laser is currently considered to be the treatment of choice for rhinophyma and actinic cheilitis because of the excellent cosmetic results that can be obtained with quicker healing times and minimized risk of scarring (15–21). Similarly, epidermal lesions, such as seborrheic keratoses, dermatosis papulosa nigra, and epidermal nevi, respond favorably to carbon dioxide laser vaporization (35). Syringomas, trichilemmomas, xanthelasma, sebaceous hyperplasia, and benign compound nevi, though dermal in nature, have also been removed successfully without complications (40–42). Finally, autologous collagen grafts can be harvested with ease from the postauricular sulcus or upper eyelid after the epidermis is vaporized with the laser beam in a defocused mode. The dermal grafts are then excised, contoured, and transplanted to the desired location (C. Weinstein, *personal communication*).

Although there are no absolute contraindications to carbon dioxide laser resurfacing, limited results may be expected in some situations. As mentioned previously, rhytides related to muscle activity (e.g., glabellar lines, forehead wrinkles, and nasolabial folds) are rarely improved permanently by any resurfacing technique but may show a variable degree of clinical improvement that can last up to several years after carbon dioxide laser treatment. Patients who have recently taken oral retinoids should not undergo laser resurfacing procedures for at least 1–2 years following cessation of their retinoid therapy, as they may have an increased risk of scarring (43). While fair-skinned patients are better candidates than patients with dark or olive skin tones, laser resurfacing can still be performed. It is important to note that prolonged hyperpigmentation can be expected post-operatively in these cases, which will eventually disappear spontaneously or with the use of hydroquinone-containing preparations. Lastly, patients who have had other forms of treatment prior to presentation which resulted in varying degrees of tissue fibrosis (i.e., dermabrasion, chemical peel, or silicone injections), may have less impressive results following laser resurfacing.

14   2.3 PREOPERATIVE EVALUATION

Patients believe that lasers are like magic wands, capable of removing every blemish without any side effects. In essence, no patient wants to be "inconvenienced" by a little bit of laser surgery. It is therefore imperative to provide patients with a realistic scenario of what can be achieved with their particular skin condition and the expected postoperative course of events. In addition, it is important to assess a patient's entire skin as, very often, patients will focus on a particular area (such as wrinkles at the upper lip) rather than noticing the presence of deep wrinkles everywhere else. In these instances, a surgeon is not helping a patient by resurfacing the perioral rhytides alone. A checklist of questions are thus particularly helpful when initially evaluating a patient for laser resurfacing (Table 2.2).

1. Does the patient have lesions that are amenable to laser resurfacing?

Patients with facial or eyelid ptosis fare better with facelifting procedures and blepharoplasties, respectively. On the other hand, lines around the lips and eyes are ideally suited for laser treatment. If movement lines (glabellar, forehead, nasolabial folds) are the primary concern, some (albeit temporary) improvement may be achieved with laser resurfacing. Widespread acne (pitted) scars can expect good results, as can epidermal and dermal lesions noted previously.

2. Does the patient have the correct skin type?

Although fair-skinned (Fitzpatrick types 1 and 2) patients are ideal for resurfacing procedures, darker-skinned individuals are also suitable. Because patients with darker skin tones tend to develop tran-

TABLE 2.2   Evaluation of a Patient for Laser Resurfacing

- Are the patient's lesions amenable to laser surgery?
- What is the patient's skin type?
- Does the patient have realistic expectations?
- Has the patient taken oral retinoids?
- Does the patient have a life-style incongruous with postsurgical activity limitations?
- Has the patient ever had cold sores?
- Does the patient have a tendency toward hypertrophic or keloid scar formation?
- Is the patient allergic to any anesthetic or topical formulation?
- Has the patient ever had another form of treatment (i.e., dermabrasion, chemical peel, facelift, blepharoplasty, silicone or collagen injections)?

sient postinflammatory hyperpigmentation, it is important to fore-warn them of this possibility.

3. Does the patient have realistic expectations?

Patients who expect to have perfectly smooth skin are poor candi-dates for *any* resurfacing procedure. Although improvement is to be expected, perfection is rarely possible to achieve. It is helpful to show patients before and after photographs of other patients who have undergone laser resurfacing for similar skin lesions. Although it is tempting to display one's best before and after photographs, it is advisable to show average results so that a patient will realize the limitations of the procedure. It is also important to reiterate to patients that the aim of laser resurfacing is to improve skin contour, not to perfect dyspigmentation or eliminate pores, as many patients have the mistaken impression that they will no longer need makeup after laser surgery.

4. Has the patient recently taken oral retinoids?

There is increasing evidence that poor healing and unpredictable scarring may occur for at least 2 years following treatment with oral retinoids. Since there is no sure way of predicting which patients are at risk for such sequelae, it is best to wait as long as possible after oral retinoid ingestion before performing resurfacing or, if possible, to perform the laser surgery *before* the patient begins retinoid treat-ment.

5. What is the patient's life-style?

Patients who either work outdoors or spend most of their recre-ational time involved in outdoor sports may find it difficult to avoid sun exposure for 2 or 3 months following the laser resurfacing pro-cedure. Although these patients need not be excluded from treat-ment, it is important to insist that they wear sunscreens on a regu-lar basis.

2.4 PATIENT INFORMATION

If the patient is deemed to be a suitable candidate for carbon diox-ide laser resurfacing, a full explanation (verbal and written) is given regarding the laser procedure, expected length of surgery, anesthe-sia used, and postoperative activity and wound care. An education-al video that outlines the procedure and postoperative course of events is very helpful and reassuring, as are before and after pho-tographs of patients with similar conditions.

Immediately following surgery, patients can return home, during which time antibiotic ointment or semipermeable dressings are applied and changed daily. Ice packs and mild analgesics are pre-

16 scribed over the first 24–48 hours. Following the initial oozing or crusting stage (lasting an average of 5 days), any residual erythema can be covered with makeup. Opaque sunscreens (containing titanium dioxide) serve as excellent primers, thereby serving a dual role. Sun protection is necessary for at least 2–3 months following laser resurfacing, as ultraviolet light can lead to irregular pigmentation during the healing phase. Any patient who has had a history of cold sores (regardless of how remote) are given acyclovir prophylactically, beginning 24 hours prior to the procedure for a total of 7–10 days (until complete reepithelialization occurs). Preoperative use of topical retinoic acid and/or glycolic acid is not routinely advised. Patients already using topical retinoids or glycolic acid preparations are allowed to continue their use preoperatively but usually do not continue during the initial postoperative stages due to excessive irritation. Patients can return to work as soon as they feel comfortable. Most prefer to wait until their laser-treated areas can be covered with makeup and any associated swelling has subsided (usually by day 7–10).

2.5 CARBON DIOXIDE LASER REJUVENATION PROCEDURE

2.5.1 Anesthesia

Depending on the type of anesthesia used (local or intravenous), patients are asked to arrive 15–30 minutes before their scheduled procedure. For those requiring intravenous sedation, patients are instructed to avoid food and drink for 6 hours prior. Patients are instructed to wear comfortable clothing and be accompanied by a friend or relative. Preoperative medications are administered and topical anesthetic cream is applied. If limited areas are being resurfaced (e.g., perioral or periorbital rhytides), local anesthesia (intralesional or nerve blocks) is used. Wrinkles are outlined with a marking pen prior to injections. In those instances when full skin resurfacing is performed, intravenous sedation (Midazolam) may be required. A pulse oximeter and cardiac monitor should be used in these latter cases. Oxygen is not usually necessary and is a hazard due to its incendiary potential.

2.5.2 Skin Preparation

Skin preparation includes a total facial scrub with aqueous chlorhexidine to remove makeup and debris. Alcoholic preparations are contraindicated due to their flammability. Hair-bearing areas are protected or dampened with wet sponges. Protective eyeshields or goggles are then placed on the patient.

2.5.3 Laser Procedure

17

Periorbital Rhytides   It is important to vaporize the skin laterally and inferiorly from the orbital rims to the furthest extent of the rhytides. The globe should be protected with a sandblasted Jaeger plate or other eyeshields and the eyelashes displaced from the operative field with the back of a water-moistened cotton swab or gauze. While laser settings will vary from one operator to the next, most surgeons use 500 mJ per pulse at 3–7 watts. The collimated 3-mm handpiece is kept perpendicular to the skin at all times. The depth of resurfacing will depend on how rapidly the laser is moved across the field. It is best to avoid overlapping laser pulses to avoid charring and subsequent tissue overheating. The entire area is resurfaced rather than limiting the laser pulses only to the areas between each rhytide ("shoulders"). After the first pass, the ablated skin (epidermis) is removed with water or saline-soaked gauze. It is important to hydrate the skin between each laser pass in order to ascertain the level of penetration and to prevent char formation. Usually with the second laser pass, dermal contraction can be clearly seen and the wrinkle line diminishes or disappears. During this pass, one can be more selective in treating the wrinkles and shoulders rather than lasing the entire area. On average, only one to two passes are required in the infraorbital region; however, two or more passes may be needed laterally where wrinkles are often deeper and the skin is thicker.

Perioral Rhytides   As with periorbital rhytides, perioral lines should be resurfaced as a whole cosmetic unit. Instead of tracing down each individual wrinkle (which can lead to depressions and unevenness), the entire upper and lower lip region is treated in a horizontal nature (perpendicular to the wrinkles) using 500 mJ per pulse and 5–10 watts. After each pass, the area is wiped with water or saline-soaked gauze and an assessment is made. Repeat laser passes are made across the wrinkle lines only until no discernible wrinkles remain. In general, two to five passes may be required, depending on the depth of the original rhytides and the thickness of the skin.

Glabellar and Forehead Lines   A similar technique is used here as with periorbital and perioral rhytides. The entire cosmetic unit is treated (usually two to five passes) with 500 mJ, 5–10 watts.

Cheeks, Chin, and Nose (Acne Scars)   Broad sweeps over the entire involved skin surface are performed without overlapping laser spots using 500 mJ and 5–10 watts. As when treating rhytides, the coagulated skin is removed after each pass with water or saline-soaked gauze and the areas are retreated until the entire surface appears regular. After the first pass, the acne scars are better defined—appearing as white, slightly depressed areas. Further passes are made around and across the scars, allowing the dermis to visibly contract around the scars. Because there is no bleeding, the treatment endpoint (relative effacement of the scars) is easily determined.

2.6 POSTOPERATIVE CARE

While some surgeons prefer semiocclusive biosynthetic dressings, others simply advise the use of topical antibiotics. In either case, keeping an area well-hydrated (occluded) promotes rapid healing and minimizes postoperative pain.

Depending on the level of resurfacing, oral antibiotics may be prescribed as prophylaxis. Acyclovir is prescribed for any patient with a history of cold sores and is continued for 10 days until reepithelialization occurs. While most patients suffer little to no pain, mild analgesics are advised. Oral prednisolone (25–100 mg daily for 5 days) can be given to minimize postoperative edema, especially when large areas have been treated.

Once the treated areas are no longer crusting, sunscreen and makeup can be applied. For those patients who develop postinflammatory hyperpigmentation (usually apparent at 1 month postoperatively), a hydroquinone-containing cream mixed with glycolic acid or retinoic acid and hydrocortisone can be applied twice daily. (See Table 2.3.)

TABLE 2.3 Laser Resurfacing Checklist

PREOPERATIVE	
Patient education	Information and instruction sheet
	Baseline photographs
	Consent form
INTRAOPERATIVE	
Anesthesia	Topical, local, tumescent, nerve block, intravenous
Skin preparation	Chlorhexidine (no alcohol!)
Eye protection	Goggles, eye shields
Laser parameters	Ultrapulse setting, 500 mJ, 3–10 watts
Other	Water or saline-soaked gauze
POSTOPERATIVE	
Home care	Semiocclusive dressings or topical antibiotics
	Ice packs
	Acetaminophen or other analgesics
	± Acyclovir, oral antibiotics, steroids
Follow-up	0.5, 1, 2, 4, 8 week examinations and photographs

2.7 SIDE EFFECTS

Fortunately, side effects are uncommon following pulsed carbon dioxide laser surgery. Erythema is usual and should not be regarded as a complication of treatment. It typically lasts 6–10 weeks and requires camouflaging with makeup. Prolonged erythema or induration may signify early hypertrophic scarring (see Chapter 8). Milia and acne may occur transiently, especially if occlusive ointments are used postoperatively. Adding retinoic or glycolic acid to the skin regimen will help to reduce or remove milia, while topical or oral antibiotics may be required for treatment of acne.

As with any surgical procedure, infection can be a complication. Should this occur, cultures should be obtained and the patient started on oral broad-spectrum antibiotics. Herpetic infections can occur in any patient with a history of cold sores despite prophylaxis with acyclovir. Continued treatment with acyclovir is advised with diligent local care.

Hyperpigmentation is not uncommon, especially in patients with deeper skin tones, but fortunately, is almost always transient. While most cases will resolve spontaneously, the use of a hydroquinone-containing preparation and avoidance of ultraviolet light can hasten the fading process.

As with all resurfacing techniques, scarring may occur if the procedure is performed too vigorously with excessive dermal penetration. In addition, the risk of scarring may be increased in patients who have recently been treated with oral retinoids or in those who develop secondary bacterial infection. Fortunately, the controlled tissue ablative properties and improved visualization of treatment endpoints using the pulsed carbon dioxide laser greatly reduce the risk of scarring or untoward collagen destruction.

2.8 SUMMARY

While continuous-wave carbon dioxide lasers have been able to successfully vaporize tissue for years, heat conduction to the surrounding skin with resultant scarring limited their use in cutaneous resurfacing. With the subsequent development of high-energy, pulsed carbon dioxide lasers, clean ablation of the skin could be achieved without significant heating of normal adjacent tissue. Thus the carbon dioxide laser has become an ideal tool for resurfacing rhytides, atrophic or pitted scars, and benign skin growths. In addition, because of their precision and lack of thermal injury, the new high-energy, pulsed carbon dioxide lasers can be used to treat lesions in previously difficult cosmetic areas, such as the perioral and periorbital areas, with minimal risk of untoward complications, such as scarring or permanent pigment alteration.

CASE 2.1 FACIAL RHYTIDES

A 52-year-old woman with extensive facial rhytides following years of ultraviolet light exposure (Case Figure 2.1A).

Anesthesia: IV Midazolam and direct infiltration of 2% lidocaine without epinephrine.

Procedure: Full face resurfacing with Coherent Ultrapulse carbon dioxide laser.

Laser Parameters: Periorbital region: 500 mJ/pulse, 3 watts, 1–2 passes, 3-mm spot size. Perioral region: 500 mJ/pulse, 10 watts, 2 passes, 3-mm spot size. Cheeks: 400 mJ/pulse, 15 watts, 1–2 passes, 3-mm spot size.

Postoperative Care: Semiocclusive dressings (Flexipore) for 1 week.

Postoperative Results: Same patient 3 months following laser treatment demonstrated marked improvement of all rhytides (Case Figure 2.1B).

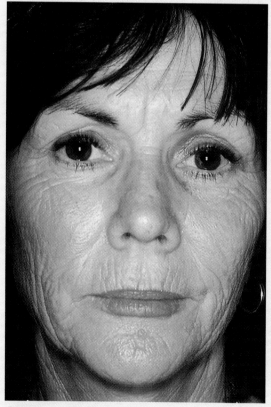
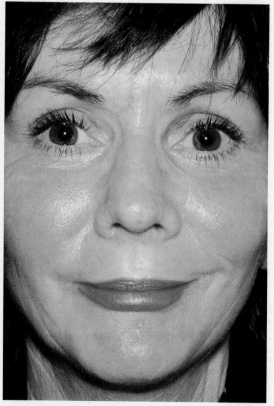

Case 2.1A Before   Case 2.1B After

CASE 2.2 PERIORBITAL RHYTIDES

A 34-year-old man with moderate periorbital rhytides (Case Figures 2.2A,B).

Anesthesia: Topical 30% lidocaine cream in velvachol base under occlusion for 30 minutes.

Procedure: Comparison study of Coherent Ultrapulse carbon dioxide laser with Surgilase Superpulse carbon dioxide system.

Laser Parameters: Right periorbital region: Ultrapulse carbon dioxide laser at 400 mJ/pulse, 5 watts, 1–2 passes, 3-mm spot size. Left periorbital region: Surgipulse carbon dioxide laser at 400 mJ/pulse, 5 watts, 3–4 passes, 3-mm spot size.

Postoperative Care: Cool water compresses and/or ice pack 2-4 times daily followed by topical antibiotic ointment and petrolatum. Acetaminophen as needed for pain.

Postoperative Results: Improvement of rhytides in both eyes was seen 8 weeks following surgery (Case Figures 2.2C,D). (*Note:* Slightly enhanced results are seen on the right side where the Ultrapulse carbon dioxide laser was used.)

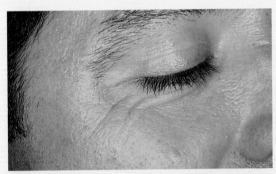

Case 2.2A Before (Right periorbit)

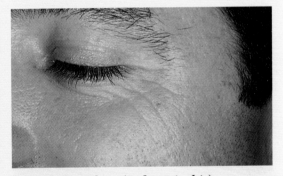

Case 2.2B Before (Left periorbit)

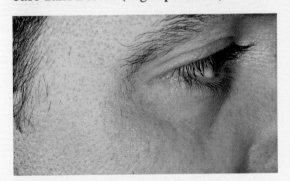

Case 2.2C After (Right periorbit)

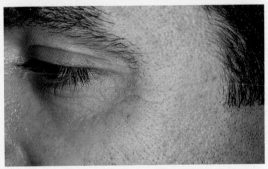

Case 2.2D After (Left periorbit)

CASE 2.3 PERIORAL RHYTIDES

A 52-year-old woman with prominent perioral rhytides (Case Figure 2.3A). No patient history of smoking but had excessive sun damage in years past. Positive history of oral HSV.

Anesthesia: Topical 30% lidocaine cream and nerve blocks of second and third branches of trigeminal nerve (V_2–V_3) using 1% lidocaine without epinephrine.

Procedure: Coherent Ultrapulse carbon dioxide laser resurfacing of perioral region.

Laser Parameters: 500 mJ/pulse, 5 watts, 3–5 passes, 3 mm spot size (Case Figure 2.3B shows wiping of tissue with saline-soaked gauze between laser passes).

Postoperative Care: Cool water compresses and/or ice every 2 hours while awake followed by topical antibiotic ointment and petrolatum for first 2 days. Twice daily application of antibiotic ointment or petrolatum thereafter until full healing. Acetominophen as needed for pain. Acyclorir 4000 mg. TID for 10 days.

Postoperative Results: Same patient 6 weeks following laser treatment showed reduction in deep rhytides (Case Figure 2.3C).

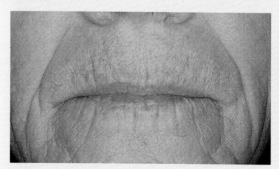

Case 2.3A Immediately before treatment

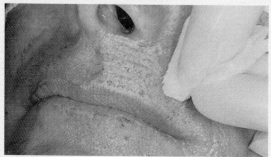

2.3B During laser treatment, char-free skin is removed with saline soaked-gauze.

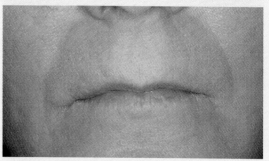

Case 2.3C 6 weeks following laser treatment

CASE 2.4 ATROPHIC ACNE SCARRING

A 32-year-old woman with extensive atrophic acne scarring of the cheeks, temples, chin, and jaw (Case Figure 2.4A).

Anesthesia: Tumescent anesthesia using 0.05% lidocaine with 1:1,000,000 epinephrine (total amount = 100–200 cc per cheek).

Procedure: Ultrapulse carbon dioxide laser resurfacing of the cheeks, chin, nose, and temples.

Laser Parameters: 400 mJ/pulse, 17 watts, 1–2 passes, 3-mm spot size.

Postoperative Care: Semiocclusive dressings (Flexipore) for 1 week.

Postoperative Results: Three months following surgery, a noticeable improvement in skin texture and degree of scarring was seen (Case Figure 2.4B).

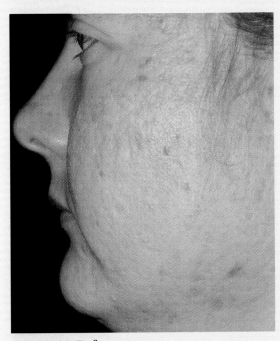

Case 2.4A Before

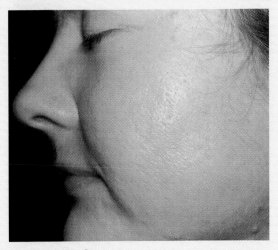

Case 2.4B After

CASE 2.5 EPIDERMAL NEVUS

A 38-year-old woman with epidermal nevus extending down right side of face (Case Figure 2.5A).

Anesthesia: Tumescent anesthesia using 0.05% lidocaine with 1:1,000,000 epinephrine (100–200 cc per cheek).

Procedure: Full face resurfacing with Coherent Ultrapulse carbon dioxide laser.

Laser Parameters: 400 mJ/pulse, 10–12 watts, 1 pass, 3-mm spot size.

Postoperative Care: Semiocclusive dressings (Flexipore) for 1 week.

Postoperative Results: Same patient 6 weeks following laser treatment showed absence of initial lesion and no dyspigmentation (Case Figure 2.5B).

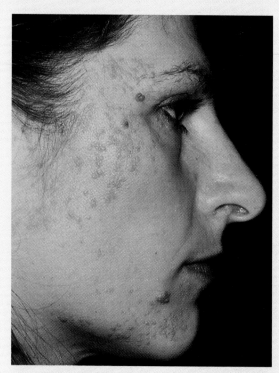

Case 2.5A Before

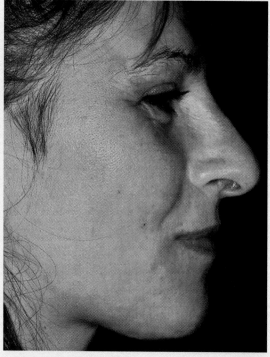

Case 2.5B After

REFERENCES

1. Maiman TH. Stimulated optical radiation in ruby. *Nature* 1960;187: 483–94.

2. Anderson RR, Parrish JA. Selective photothermolysis: precise micro-surgery by selective absorption of pulsed radiation. *Science* 1983;22:524–7.

3. Anderson RR, Parrish JA. Microvasculature can be selectively damaged using dye lasers: a basic theory and experimental evidence in human skin. *Lasers Surg Med* 1981;1:263–76.

4. Parrish JA, Anderson RR, Harris T, Paul B, Murphy GF. Selective thermal effects with pulsed irradiation from lasers: from organ to organelle. *J Invest Dermatol* 1983;80(suppl):75–80.

5. Tan OT, Sherwood K, Gilchrest BA. Treatment of children with port–wine stains using the flashlamp-pulsed tunable dye laser. *N Engl J Med* 1989;320:416–21.

6. Alster TS, Tan OT. Laser treatment of benign cutaneous vascular lesions. *Am Fam Physician* 1991;44:547–54.

7. Ashinoff R, Geronemus RG. Flashlamp–pumped pulsed dye laser for port–wine stains in infancy: earlier versus later treatment. *J Am Acad Dermatol* 1991;24:467–72.

8. Goldman MP, Fitzpatrick RE, Ruiz–Esparza J. Treatment of port–wine stains (capillary malformation) with the flashlamp–pumped pulsed dye laser. *J Pediatr* 1993;122:71–7.

9. Alster TS, Wilson F. Treatment of port–wine stains with the flash-lamp–pumped pulsed dye laser: extended clinical experience in children and adults. *Ann Plast Surg* 1994;32:478–84.

10. Slutzki S, Shafir R, Bornstein LA. Use of the carbon dioxide laser for large excisions with minimal blood loss. *Plast Reconstr Surg* 1977;60:250–255.

11. Baker SS, Muenzler WS, Small RG, Leonard JE. Carbon dioxide laser blepharoplasty. *Ophthalmology* 1984;91:238–43.

12. Wesley RE, Bond JB. Carbon dioxide laser in ophthalmic plastic and orbital surgery. *Ophthal Surg* 1985;18:631–3.

13. David LM. The laser approach to blepharoplasty. *J Dermatol Surg Oncol* 1988;14:741–6.

14. Morrow DM, Morrow LB. Carbon dioxide laser blepharoplasty. *J Dermatol Surg Oncol* 1992;18:307–13.

15. Shapshay SM, Strong MS, Anastasi GW, et al. Removal of rhinophyma with the carbon dioxide laser. A preliminary report. *Arch Otolaryngol* 1980;106:257–9.

16. Greenbaum SS, Krull EA, Watnick K. Comparison of CO_2 laser and electrosurgery in the treatment of rhinophyma. *J Am Acad Dermatol* 1988;18:363–368.

17. Wheeland RG, Bailin PL, Ratz JL. Combined carbon dioxide laser excision and vaporization in the treatment of rhinophyma. *J Dermatol Surg Oncol* 1987;13:172–177.

18. David LM. Laser vermillion ablation for actinic cheilitis. *J Dermatol Surg Oncol* 1985;11:605–608.

26

19. Whitaker DC. Microscopically proven cure of actinic cheilitis by CO_2 laser. *Lasers Surg Med* 1987;7:520–3.

20. Dufresne RG Jr, Garrett AB, Bailin PL, Ratz JL. Carbon dioxide laser treatment of chronic actinic cheilitis. *J Am Acad Dermatol* 1988;19:876–8.

21. Stanley RJ, Roenick RK. Actinic cheilitis—treatment with the carbon dioxide laser. *Mayo Clin Proc* 1988;63:230–235.

22. David LM, Sanders GH. Carbon dioxide laser blepharoplasty. A comparison to cold steel and electrocautery. *J Dermatol Surg Oncol* 1987;13:110–4.

23. Mittleman HM, Apfelberg DB. Carbon dioxide laser blepharoplasty—advantages and disadvantages. *Ann Plast Surg* 1990;24:1–6.

24. Wentzell JM, Robinson JK, Wentzell JM Jr, Schwartz DE, Carlson SE. Physical properties of aerosols produced by dermabrasion. *Arch Dermatol* 1989;125:1637–1643.

25. Brody HJ. Variations and comparisons in medium depth chemical peeling. *J Dermatol Surg Oncol* 1989;15:953–63.

26. Hobbs ER, Bailin PC, Wheeland RG, Ratz JL. Superpulsed lasers: minimizing thermal damage with short duration, high irradiance pulses. *J Dermatol Surg Oncol* 1987;13:955–64.

27. Deckelbaum LI, Isner JM, Donaldson RF, Laliberte SM, Clark RH, Salerm DN. Use of pulsed energy delivery to minimize tissue injury resulting from CO_2 laser irradiation of cardiovascular tissues. *J Am Coll Cardiol* 1986;7:898–900.

28. Lanzafame RJ, Naim JO, Rogers DW, Hinshaw R. Comparison of continuous wave, shop–wave and superpulse laser wounds. *Lasers Surg Med* 1988;8:119–24.

29. Walsh JT, Flotte TJ, Anderson RR, Deutsch TF. Pulsed CO_2 laser tissue ablation: effect of tissue type and pulse duration on thermal damage. *Lasers Surg Med* 1989;8:108–18.

30. Walsh JT, Deutsch TF. Pulsed CO_2 laser ablation: measurement of the ablation rate. *Lasers Surg Med* 1988;8:264–75.

31. Fitzpatrick RE, Ruiz–Esparza J, Goldman MP. The depth of thermal necrosis using the CO_2 laser: a comparison of the superpulsed mode and conventional mode. *J Dermatol Surg Oncol* 1991;17:340–4.

32. Zweig AD, Meierhofer B, Muller OM, Mischler C, Romano V, Frenz M, Weber HP. Lateral thermal damage along pulsed laser incisions. *Lasers Surg Med* 1990;10:262–74.

33. Schomacker KT, Walsh JT, Flotte TJ, Deutsch TF. Thermal damage produced by high–irradiance continuous wave CO_2 laser cutting of tissue. *Lasers Surg Med* 1990;10:74–84.

34. Fuller TA. Laser tissue interaction: the influence of power density. In: Baggish MS, ed. *Basic and advanced laser surgery in gynecology.* Norwalk CT: Appleton–Century–Crofts, 1985.

35. Fitzpatrick RE, Goldman MP, Ruiz–Esparza J. Clinical advantage of the CO_2 laser superpulsed mode. Treatment of verruca vulgaris, seborrheic keratoses, lentigines, and actinic cheilitis. *J Dermatol Surg Oncol* 1994;20:449–56.

36. Weinstein C. Ultrapulse carbon dioxide laser removal of periocular wrinkles in association with laser blepharoplasty. *J Clin Laser Med Surg* 1994;12:205–9.

37. Alster TS. Comparison of the superpulse CO_2 and ultrapulse CO_2 lasers in the treatment of periorbital rhytides. *Dermatol Surg (in press)*.

38. Alster TS, Garg S. Treatment of facial rhytides with the ultrapulse high-energy carbon dioxide laser. *Plast Reconstr Surg (in press)*.

39. Alster TS, West TB. Resurfacing of atrophic facial scars with a high-energy, pulsed carbon dioxide laser. *Dermatol Surg (in press)*.

40. Wheeland RG, McGillis ST. Cowden's disease—treatment of cutaneous lesions using carbon dioxide laser vaporization: a comparison of conventional and superpulsed techniques. *J Dermatol Surg Oncol* 1989;15:1055–9.

41. Apfelberg DB, Maser MR, Lash H, White DN, Cosman B. Superpulse CO_2 laser treatment of facial syringomata. *Lasers Surg Med* 1987;7:533–7.

42. Alster TS, West TB. Ultrapulse CO_2 laser ablation of xanthelasma. *J Am Acad Dermatol (in press)*.

43. Rubenstein R, Roenick HH, Stegan SJ, Hanke CW. Atypical keloids after dermabrasion of patients taking isotretinoin. *J Am Acad Dermatol* 1986;15:280–285.

3

LASER-ASSISTED BLEPHAROPLASTY AND MELOPLASTY

David B. Apfelberg, M.D.

3.1 INTRODUCTION

Facial cosmetic surgery has been enhanced with the addition of lasers. Two laser systems, in particular, have emerged as being the most useful. Initially, the carbon dioxide laser was utilized in blepharoplasty surgery and, later, for facelifting procedures as well. More recently, the YAG laser at 1064 nm and the KTP frequency-doubled YAG laser at 532 nm have been reported to be useful in these same procedures.

3.2 BACKGROUND STUDIES

Several authors have investigated and compared wound healing using the carbon dioxide and YAG lasers versus conventional scalpel surgery. Hambley et al. (1) showed, using animal and microscopic studies, that more damage to the skin resulted from the standard carbon dioxide laser incision as compared to scalpel incisions on the basis of clinical evaluation, histopathology of reepithelialization, and measurement of tensile strength. Norris and Mullarkey (2) compared incisions made by the scalpel and the carbon dioxide laser in hog skin and found no difference at 30 days, although the initial reepithelialization and tensile strength were diminished in the car-

Cosmetic Laser Surgery, Edited by Alster, M.D. and Apfelberg, M.D.
ISBN 0471-12242-4 © 1996 Wiley-Liss, Inc.

30

bon dioxide laser incision in the first 2 weeks. Mittelman et al. (3) studied facial skin incised by scalpel, by cautery, and by carbon dioxide, KTP frequency-doubled YAG (532 nm), and standard (1064 nm) YAG lasers. They concluded that the acute stage of healing demonstrated greater tissue injury from lasers and cautery. Mean tensile strength of cautery and laser wounds were later studied by Dickson et al. (4), who found decreased tensile strength in these wounds when compared to scalpel excision at 2 weeks, but equal and better tensile strength of laser and scalpel wounds compared to cautery at 4 weeks. Thus although lasers were found to be more hemostatic than scalpel excisions, they appeared to cause excessive epithelial and dermal injury during the initial stages of wound healing.

The development of the carbon dioxide laser blepharoplasty was preceded by the use of lasers for a variety of ocular and adnexal lesions. In 1980, Beckman et al. (5) described numerous uses for lasers in ocular surgery (i.e.,glaucoma, scleral diseases) and adnexal lesions (i.e., hemangiomas, lid tumors). Wesley and Bond (6) also described the use of the carbon dioxide laser for lymphangiomas, hemangiomas, and anticoagulated patients. Korn and Glotzbach (7) repaired medial ectropion by carbon dioxide laser resection of conjunctiva and tarsus-inferior muscle.

The use of the carbon dioxide laser for blepharoplasty was initially reported by Baker and colleagues in 1984 (8). Of the 40 patients followed an average of 16 months, it was apparent that the carbon dioxide laser improved intraoperative hemorrhage and postoperative ecchymosis and edema. Baker subsequently updated his experience in 1992 and described the use of the David–Baker clamp for protection of the eye and retraction of tissue during the laser procedure (9). David and Sanders, in contralateral comparison studies, reported better results on the side treated with the carbon dioxide laser than on the side treated with a scalpel/cautery procedure (10). Carbon dioxide laser techniques, including the transconjunctival lower blepharoplasty approach, were further described by David (11,12), Trelles et al. (13), and Spadoni and Cain (14). Morrow and Morrow (15) compared laser blepharoplasty with conventional blepharoplasty in a contralateral study of ten patients and concluded that the laser reduced operating time, bleeding, bruising, swelling, and postoperative pain due to the shorter recovery time. Mittelman and Apfelberg (16) were not able to demonstrate significant differences between laser-assisted and traditional blepharoplasty; however, they did not use the laser as extensively during the procedure, thereby limiting direct comparisons with other similar studies. Beeson et al. (17) noted that the superpulsed carbon dioxide laser produced less bruising and swelling as a result of decreased operative time when compared with contralateral scalpel/cautery surgery, especially when the surgeon was experienced in the use of the laser. In 1992, Morrow and Morrow (18) reported on a series of

110 lower facelifts using the carbon dioxide laser as the only cutting instrument and found less postoperative bruising, swelling, and pain.

Several reports have detailed the use of the contact YAG laser in facial cosmetic surgery. In 1990, Putterman (19) reported the results of a 3-year study of 18 oculoplastic patients, 10 of whom underwent contralateral procedures comparing laser to conventional surgery. The laser side demonstrated less bleeding, operative time, and pain during fat resection, but postoperative ecchymosis and edema were not significantly different from that resulting with scalpel surgery. The advantages of the YAG laser in plastic surgery has best been documented for the removal of hemangiomas and other tumors. In 1989, Apfelberg et al. (20) described the use of sapphire tip technology for YAG laser excisions of hemangiomas, lymphangiomas, neurofibromas, and hamartomas with excellent hemostasis. Further reports by Apfelberg and colleagues (21–23) have shown the benefit of the YAG laser in the resection of massive cavernous hemangiomas with less blood loss and increased safety margins.

Given the clear advantages of hemostatic control obtained with the use of the YAG laser, application of the same laser techniques was a natural for delicate facial cosmetic procedures, such as blepharoplasties and meloplasties. If equivalent hemostasis could be achieved, the patient could benefit from diminished blood loss, bruising, swelling, pain, and recovery time. Keller (24) documented less bleeding and greater visualization during surgery as well as reduced bruising and swelling during recovery following use of the KTP frequency-doubled YAG laser for face, eye, and forehead lifts. More recently, Apfelberg (25) reported his experience with 9 facelift and 19 blepharoplasty patients using the YAG laser with contact sapphire tips. Bleeding, bruising, and swelling were dimished by one-third (average of 11 days for laser versus 17 days for conventional surgery) in the contralateral study cases with an estimated blood loss of only 7.7 cc in blepharoplasty patients.

3.3 DESCRIPTION OF YAG LASER PROCEDURE

The YAG laser (Heraeus Laser Sonics Hercules Model 5040) is utilized with 10–15 watts of power transmitted through fiber optics to a frosted sapphire tip of 0.6–0.8 mm diameter. Either a continuous wave mode is used for cutting with coagulation on the face or a lower power (5–8 watts) mode with 0.01 second pulse and 0.01-second interval is used for more gentle treatment on the eyelids. Skin incision with the laser always produces a narrow zone of thermal necrosis [reported experimentally to be as small as 50–200 micrometers (μm)], which is best resected with fine scissors or scalpel prior to closure for prevention of scar formation or wound dehiscence.

The sapphire tip is carbonized by application to a dry tongue blade to produce a short burning. This prepares the tip for immediate incision when applied to the skin.

3.4 DESCRIPTION OF ULTRAPULSE CARBON DIOXIDE LASER PROCEDURE

The Coherent Ultrapulse 5000 carbon dioxide laser is used in the "ultrapulsed" mode. To achieve the higher powers than would normally be possible if the laser were operated on a continuous-wave (CW) or superpulsed mode, the laser tube is supercharged with high doses of radiofrequency energy for a very short time (pulse). The Ultrapulse can thus achieve high power over one-millionth of a second. The pulses may be repeated at a certain repetition rate (pulse per second equals hertz). Laser settings that would yield an average power of 5 watts include a repetition rate of 25 hertz (Hz), a pulse width of 314 microseconds (μs), and energy per pulse of 250 millijoules (mJ). The clinical result is skin vaporization or incision without char or excessive thermal injury to tissue. Since the thermal relaxation time of skin is established to be approximately 695–700 μs, the short pulse does not allow accumulation of heat. Also, the delay between pulses permits the minimal level of heat that has accumulated in surrounding areas to dissipate before the next burst of laser energy is delivered. The result is extremely precise vaporization or cutting with minimal risk of scarring or prolonged healing time from unwanted thermal damage. The Ultrapulse carbon dioxide laser thus represents a significant advance over previous continuous wave carbon dioxide laser technology, because it comes close to achieving a "cold incision."

The laser handpiece is held at the focal length and directed toward tissue that is placed on traction for easier separation. Prior to tissue application, the laser is directed toward a moistened tongue blade to check alignment. Utilizing 3–5 watts of power, 25–50 mJ, and a 0.2-mm spot size, excellent hemostatic cutting may be achieved. Skin, subcutaneous tissue, fat, and muscle are easily incised. Defocusing the laser beam permits coagulation. Since there is little or no adjacent tissue thermal damage, it is not necessary to cut back wound edges prior to closure as with the YAG laser.

3.5 MELOPLASTY AND BLEPHAROPLASTY WITH LASER

Facelift flaps can be undermined easily and almost bloodlessly for a distance of 3–5 cm with one exception—transection of large lumen superficial temporal vessels. Deeper or longer flap undermining is aided by injection and distention of multiple adjacent tunnels with a 14-gauge spatula tip needle and local anesthesia with epinephrine. The separations between the injected tunnels are then connected with the laser. Care is taken to keep the dissection at the proper level and to avoid "button-holing" the skin. Platysma and superficial muscular aponeurotic system (SMAS) dissection may be performed with the laser providing a bloodless field for proper observation of important anatomical structures such as facial nerves and muscles. No stimulation of the facial nerve, as seen with electrocautery, results from laser contact. Frequently, no further hemostasis is required after laser dissection. Flap advancement and closure are identical to standard facelift techniques.

Eyelid surgery is performed in a similar manner with some minor modifications. Protective eye shields are inserted over the globes after application of ophthalmic anesthetic and antibiotic ointments and are removed immediately following the procedure to prevent corneal edema. Skin, muscle, and fat may all be resected with the laser without the necessity for cross-clamping or crushing of these structures. Blood loss frequently is reported at 0–5 cc for all four lids. Transconjunctival blepharoplasty may be accomplished safely and bloodlessly as well. The laser has no electrical potential so fat may be draped directly across a small metal retractor and removed without fear of electric transmission and burning of the skin. Moistened applicators should be used as a "backstop" behind tissue that is elevated for removal by the carbon dioxide laser so that the beam will not strike tissue beyond the area to be removed. Since the YAG laser is "contact" and used as a scalpel, this precaution is not necessary.

3.6 STUDY ANALYSIS

Since 1991, 65 blepharoplasty patients, 19 combination meloplasty/blepharoplasty patients, and 1 meloplasty patient have undergone surgery utilizing either the YAG laser scalpel or the Ultrapulse carbon dioxide laser (Table 3.1). There were 8 men and 77 women, with

TABLE 3.1 Study Summary

PROCEDURE	NUMBER OF PATIENTS	SEX	AVERAGE AGE (YEARS)	BLOOD LOSS (CC)	HEALING TIME (DAYS)
Blepharoplasty	65	4 men, 61 women	48.5	7.7	11.6
Blepharoplasty/ meloplasty	19	4 men, 15 women	62.2	160	12.6
Meloplasty	1	1 woman	48	130	12.0

an average age of 48.5 years (blepharoplasty) and 62.2 years (meloplasty). Use of the lasers did not significantly lengthen or shorten the surgical procedures and there were no laser-related complications.

The results of this study were very encouraging. Postoperative swelling, ecchymosis, and pain were markedly reduced in all patients. Some patients examined at 1 day postoperative exhibited very little bruising and swelling (Case 3.1). Some patients were completely free of residual ecchymosis and swelling after 1 week. The average number of days for bruising and swelling to totally disappear without residual was 12.4 (range 4–23 days) in blepharoplasty patients and 12.6 (range 11–16 days) for meloplasty patients. SMAS dissection was enhanced by laser use with excellent hemostasis allowing for better visualization of tissue planes. Average blood loss for laser meloplasty patients was 160 cc. In approximately one-third of the blepharoplasty cases, blood loss of less than 5 cc for all four lids was recorded. Blood loss for the entire blepharoplasty group averaged 7.7 cc. Five percent of patients did not require use of any analgesic agents. Seventy-five percent of blepharoplasty patients who had laser surgery of one eyelid and standard excision of the contralateral eyelid demonstrated resolution of bruising and swelling 3–5 days earlier on the laser-treated side (Case 3.2). Many patients were able to resume normal work or social activities in 7–10 days as compared to 14–21 days for conventional procedures.

3.7 SUMMARY

The use of lasers has been shown to facilitate facial cosmetic procedures and enhance the results obtained in the immediate postoperative period (Table 3.2). Patients experience less blood loss during laser-assisted surgery with subsequent reduction in ecchymosis and edema. Contralateral studies have demonstrated that the recovery period is shortened by 30% in laser cases (7–11 days for laser-assisted surgery versus 14–17 days for standard scalpel surgery). Patients can thus return to their usual activities sooner. In addition, many patients experience little or no pain following the laser procedure, eliminating the need for prolonged analgesic use. By 3 weeks, no significant difference can be detected between contralateral treatment sides (laser versus excision). The improved hemostasis achieved with the use of the laser allows improved visualization so that vital structures can be dissected in a relatively bloodless environment.

Disadvantages of laser-assisted blepharoplasties and meloplasties include higher procedural costs. In addition, laser equipment setup and training may be too cumbersome for many practices. Laser-assisted surgeries are therefore best suited for those situations when patients require decreased time to healing (due to schedule limita-

TABLE 3.2 Advantages/Disadvantages of Laser-Assisted
Cosmetic Surgery

ADVANTAGES
- Improved hemostasis (better visualization during surgery)
- Accelerated patient recovery (diminished postoperative ecchymosis, edema, pain)
- Quicker return to daily activities postoperatively

DISADVANTAGES
- Increased procedure cost
- Cumbersome initial equipment set-up
- Special procedural and safety training requirements for physician and staff
- Potential equipment malfunction with possible revenue loss

tions) or in those patients who have a history of a coagulation disorder, are taking chronic anti-inflammatory agents, or have impaired wound healing. While cutaneous healing, scar formation, and total procedural time do not appear to be enhanced with the addition of lasers, the distinct intraoperative and early postoperative advantages clearly argue for their use in cosmetic surgery. Of course, it remains imperative to exercise one's surgical judgment in regard to patient selection, tissue resection, closure techniques, postoperative care, and follow-up examinations.

CASE 3.1 HOODED EYELIDS AND FAT HERNIATIONS

A 49-year-old female complained of sagging skin and eyelids, which had been worsening over several years (Case Figure 3.1A). No prior cosmetic procedures had been performed.

Diagnosis: Moderate hooding of the upper eyelid skin with large medial fat herniations of the upper and lower eyelids. Facial elastosis with mild jowling.

Procedure: A facelift and upper and lower transconjunctival blepharoplasties were performed under general anesthesia as an outpatient. The Ultrapulse carbon dioxide laser was used at 3 watts, 1-mm spot size, and 25 mJ. Estimated blood loss was less than 25 cc.

Postoperative Results: Mild swelling and ecchymoses were evident 1 day postoperatively (Case Figure 3.1B). By day 5, the majority of swelling and bruising had resolved (Case Figure 3.1C) and eyelid sutures were removed. Normal activities were resumed at approximately 12–14 days postoperatively (Case Figure 3.1D).

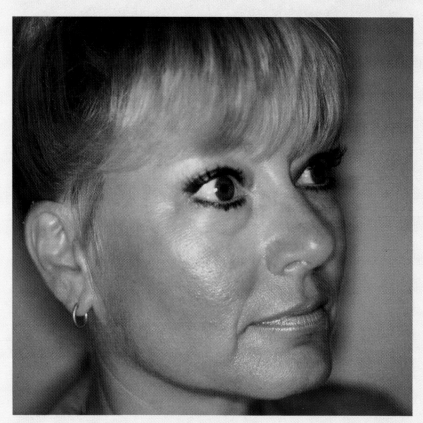

Case 3.1A Before

Postoperative Results: Mild swelling and ecchymoses were evident 1 day postoperatively (Case Figure 3.1B). By day 5, the majority of swelling and bruising had resolved (Case Figure 3.1C) and eyelid sutures were removed. Normal activities were resumed at approximately 12–14 days postoperatively (Case Figure 3.1D).

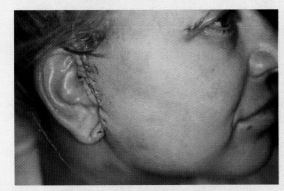

Case 3.1B One day postoperative

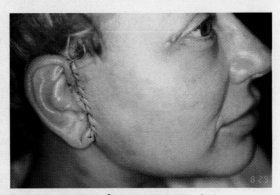

Case 3.1C Five days postoperative

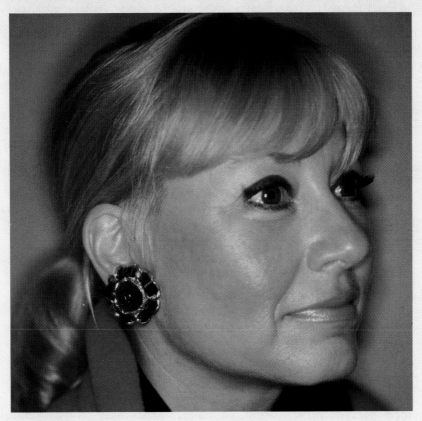

Case 3.1D After

CASE 3.2 MODERATE BLEPHAROCHALASIS AND FAT HERNIATIONS

A 34-year-old woman complained of "droopy eyelids" (Case Figure 3.2A).

Diagnosis: Moderate blepharochalasis of upper eyelids and fat herniations in upper and lower lids.

Procedure: The patient was enrolled in the experimental laser protocol in which one eye was treated with laser-assisted blepharoplasty techniques and the contralateral eye was treated using conventional scalpel techniques. The patient was unaware of which treatment was used on each side. Local anesthesia was obtained with 2% xylocaine/1:200,000 epinephrine and 0.25% marcaine/1:200,000 epinephrine. The left upper and lower eyelid received YAG laser treatment with a 0.6-mm frosted sapphire tip at 12 watts of continuous power and 3750 joules. The procedure on the right upper and lower lids was accomplished with scalpel, scissors, and cautery. Excison of skin, orbicularis muscle, and fat herniations was performed on the upper eyelids bilaterally. A transconjunctival approach for removal of fat herniations was accomplished. Approximately 5 cc of blood were lost on the left (laser) side compared to 25 cc of estimated blood loss on the right (conventional) side.

Postoperative Results: Postoperatively, the patient exhibited reduced swelling, ecchymosis, and pain on the laser-treated side. Examination at 4 days (Case Figure 3.2B) revealed more swelling as well as subconjunctival hemorrhage on the right (conventionally treated) side. Total healing of the left (laser-treated) side without residual swelling or discoloration was noted by day 9 postoperative (Case Figure 3.2C), whereas the right side required 14 days for complete healing. At 3 weeks, the patient displayed an excellent cosmetic result on both sides (Case Figure 3.2D).

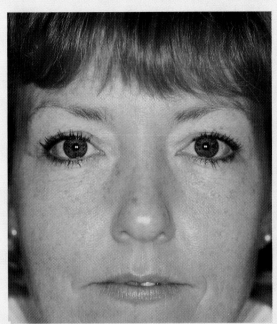

Case 3.2A Before

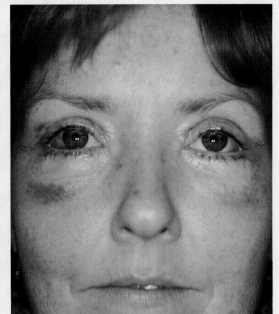

Case 3.2B Four days postoperative

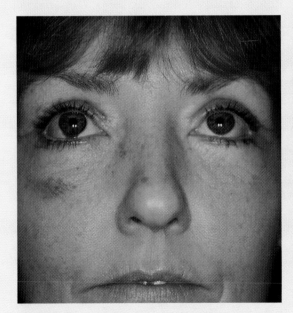

Case 3.2C Nine days postoperative

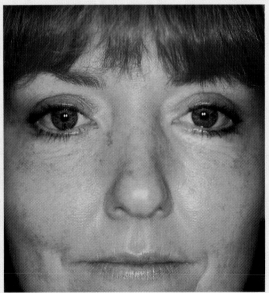

Case 3.2D After

Reprinted with permission: *Aesthetic Plastic Surgery* 1995; 231–5.

REFERENCES

1. Hambley R, Hebda P, Abell E, et al. Wound healing of skin incisions produced by ultrasonically vibrating knife, scalpel, electrosurgery and carbon dioxide laser. *J Dermatol Surg Oncol* 1988;14:1213–7.
2. Norris CW, Mullarky MB. Experimental skin incisions made with the carbon dioxide laser. *Laryngoscope* 1982;92:416–9.
3. Mittelman H, Keating W, Smoller BR. Evaluation of acute human tissue injury using various lasers in facial surgery. *Facial Plast Surg Clin North Am* 1988;173–9.
4. Dickson JB, Flanagan JC, Federman JL. Contact Nd:YAG laser. *Ophthal Plast Reconstr Surg* 1989;5:17–26.
5. Beckman H, Fuller TA, Boyman R, et al. Carbon dioxide laser surgery of the eye and adnexa. *Ophthalmology* 1980;87:999–1000.
6. Wesley RE, Bond JB. Carbon dioxide laser in ophthalmic plastic and orbital surgery. *Ophthalmic Surg* 1985;18:631–3.
7. Korn EL, Glotzpach RK. Carbon dioxide laser in ophthalmic plastic and orbital surgery. *Ophthalmic Surg* 1988;19:653–7.
8. Baker SS, Muenzler WS, Small RG, Leonard JE. Carbon dioxide laser blepharoplasty. *Ophthalmology* 1984;91:238–43.
9. Baker SS. Carbon dioxide laser upper lid blepharoplasty. *Am J Cosmetic Surg* 1992;9:141–5.
10. David LM, Sanders G. Carbon dioxide laser blepharoplasty: a comparison to cold steel and electro-cautery. *J Dermatol Surg Oncol* 1987;13:110–4.
11. David LM. The laser approach to blepharoplasty. *J Dermatol Surg Oncol* 1988;1:741–6.
12. David LM, Abergel RP. Carbon dioxide laser blepharoplasty: conjunctival temperature during surgery. *J Dermatol Surg Oncol* 1989;15:421–3.
13. Trelles MA, Sanchez J, Sala P, Elspas S. Surgical removal of lower eyelid fat using the carbon dioxide laser. *Am J Cosmetic Surg* 1992;9:149–52.
14. Spadoni D, Cain CL. Laser blepharoplasty. *AORN J* 1988;47:1184–93.
15. Morrow DM, Morrow LB. Carbon dioxide laser blepharoplasty. *J Dermatol Surg Oncol* 1992;18:307–13.
16. Mittelman HM, Apfelberg DB. Carbon dioxide laser blepharoplasty—advantages and disadvantages. *Ann Plast Surg* 1990;24:1–6.
17. Beeson WM, Kabaker S, Keller GS. Carbon dioxide laser blepharoplasty: a comparison to electrosurgery. *Int J Aesth Restor Surg* 1994;2:33–6.
18. Morrow DM, Morrow LB. Carbon dioxide laser assisted lower facellift: a preliminary report. *Am J Cosmetic Surg* 1992;9:159–68.
19. Putterman AM. Scalpel Nd:YAG laser in oculoplasty surgery. *Am J Ophthalmol* 1990;109:581–4.
20. Apfelberg DB, Maser MR, Lash H, White DN. Sapphire tip technology for YAG laser excisions in plastic surgery. *Plast Reconstr Surg* 1989;84:273–9.
21. Apfelberg DB, Maser MR, Lash H, White DN, Lane B, Marks MP. Benefits of contact and noncontact YAG laser for periorbital hemangiomas. *Ann Plast Surg* 1990;24:397–408.

22. Apfelberg DB, Lane B, Marks MP. Combined (team) approach to hemangiomas management: arteriography with superselective embolization plus YAG laser/sapphire tip resection. *Plast Reconstr Surg* 1991;88:71–82.
23. Apfelberg DB, Maser MR, Lash H, White DN, Lane B, Marks MP. Combination treatment for massive cavernous hemangiomas of the face. *Lasers Surg Med* 1990;10:217–23.
24. Keller GS. Use of the KTP laser in cosmetic surgery. *Am J Cosmetic Surg* 1992;9:177–80.
25. Apfelberg DB. YAG laser meloplasty and blepharoplasty. *Aesth Plast Surg* (*in press*).

4

SUPRAFIBROMUSCULAR AND ENDOSCOPIC RHYTIDECTOMY WITH THE HIGH-OUTPUT CARBON DIOXIDE LASER AND FLEXIBLE WAVEGUIDE

Gregory S. Keller, M.D.

4.1 INTRODUCTION

New high-energy pulsed carbon dioxide lasers produce high-energy laser beams that cut with excellent coagulation and negligible char. Delivery devices that utilize an extremely thin (0.8-mm) flexible waveguide can accurately deliver this energy to the depths of a surgical dissection. This combination of accurate fiber delivery, rapid char-free cutting, and excellent coagulation enhance the procedures of endoscopic rhytidectomy and composite and conventional rhytidectomy.

4.2 BACKGROUND

4.2.1 Pulsed Carbon Dioxide Lasers

Carbon dioxide laser light is invisible, with a wavelength in the far-infrared range of the electromagnetic spectrum (10,600 nm). This wavelength of light is strongly absorbed by tissue water and, therefore, has a shallow penetration in skin and subcutaneous tissue. When the laser light is absorbed by tissue water, vaporization of the tissue results.

Cosmetic Laser Surgery, Edited by Alster, M.D. and Apfelberg, M.D.
ISBN 0471-12242-4 © 1996 Wiley-Liss, Inc.

44

Because of its shallow penetration into tissue, the carbon dioxide laser system is a relatively precise surgical instrument, favored by surgeons in the fields of otolaryngology, plastic surgery, gynecology, and neurosurgery. However, several shortcomings of this laser have limited its usefulness in rhytidectomy surgery: (a) its lack of a fiber delivery system to accurately direct the laser energy into the depths of a surgical field, (b) its tendency to produce char when used as a cutting instrument, and (c) its diminished ability to coagulate as compared to other lasers.

Conventional carbon dioxide laser energy (joules, J) is usually described in terms of power (watts) and power density (watts/cm^2) delivered over a period of time (joules = watts × time in seconds). As the amount of power or power density that is delivered to tissue is increased, the penetrance through tissue and vaporization of tissue are also increased. Unfortunately, with conventional carbon dioxide laser systems, there is a forward and side scatter of energy so that, around the area of vaporization, a zone of coagulative necrosis and char results.

With advancements in laser technology, engineers have produced carbon dioxide lasers that are able to produce great amounts of energy in extremely short pulses (pulsed carbon dioxide lasers). These pulses are so brief that they do not exceed the thermal relaxation time of skin. Thermal relaxation is the time in which one-half of the laser heat is dissipated in the targeted skin [approximately 1 millisecond (ms)]. If the tissue relaxation time is not exceeded, the laser energy will be retained in the target tissue and the forward and side scatter of heat will be limited. The zone of necrosis will also be limited and char will not be produced. On the other hand, if the thermal relaxation time is exceeded, the excess heat produced in the target tissue could lead to scarring.

The Surgilase XJ laser delivers pulse pairs that summate to 400 millijoules (mJ). Each component of the pulse pair is less than the thermal relaxation time of skin. In contrast, the "superpulse" delivered by conventional carbon dioxide laser systems rarely exceeded 70 mJ. Because the Surgilase XJ (in its pulsed mode) delivers its energy in preset 250–400-mJ bursts, laser power (watts) is increased by delivering more bursts in a given period of time. Power (watts) can then be thought of as a delivery rate of energy (joules) or watts = joules/second. As the delivery rate of energy (watts) increases, the number of laser bursts or pulses increases (pulse rate × joules = watts) and the penetrance through tissue increases in a char-free fashion (pulse rate = watts/joules).

4.2.2 Flexible Waveguides

Carbon dioxide lasers currently cannot be delivered through a quartz fiber. As a result, the laser beam is customarily bounced off mirrors contained in a long tube with articulations (articulating arm) to a handpiece containing a lens that focuses the beam to a point (focusing handpiece). The disadvantages of the focusing hand-piece/articulating arm delivery system are (a) that the beam produced is "gaussian," having a central "hot" spot with a fall-off of energy around the edges of the beam, and (b) that the beam is difficult to focus into a surgical "hole."

Flexible waveguides transmit the waveform down the waveguide similar to the way in which a quartz fiber transmits the beam. The laser beam emerges at the target surface and may be used in an almost "contact" fashion, despite being angled in almost any direction. This is in contrast to solid tubes, which must have the beam aligned precisely down the unbendable solid tube. These flexible waveguides have a diameter as small as 0.8 mm as compared to the smaller 0.6-mm size of a quartz fiber. Because of their small diameters, they can be placed within even a very small surgical hole.

4.2.3 Other Laser Systems

Both the KTP laser (532-nm wavelength) and the Nd:YAG laser (1064-nm wavelength) have been used for rhytidectomy. Both systems utilize quartz fibers to deliver the laser beam to the tissue. The KTP laser uses a sharpened quartz fiber that tapers to 0.1 mm, "focusing" the beam down to a tiny spot. The Nd:YAG laser uses either a sharpened fiber or a sapphire tip, which again "focuses" the beam down to 0.1 or 0.2 mm. The fiber delivery systems of these lasers may be placed in direct contact with tissue.

One disadvantage of these lasers is that they cause more heat than the pulsed carbon dioxide laser systems. Because of this, they require greater skill on the part of the operator in order to avoid "button-holing" skin, especially in delicate or thin tissue areas. The increased heat disadvantage may become an advantage in male patients where there is thicker skin and where increased heat is needed for better hemostasis. The problem of increased heat may be ameliorated by the recent electronic shuttering of one of these instruments (Laserscope) to 1-ms repetitive pulses.

Another disadvantage of the KTP and Nd:YAG lasers is that they require special protective eyewear. This eyewear is colored and can be an annoyance for the surgeon to wear. Newer eyewear that is clear may serve to overcome this problem.

4.3 LASER-ASSISTED PROCEDURAL GUIDELINES

4.3.1 Flap Elevation

With the pulsed carbon dioxide laser system, a 50-mm focusing handpiece (0.1-mm laser spot) is used to make the incisions. The epidermis and upper dermis are scored in the incision line with the knife, and the incision is completed with the laser. The skin is then

46

elevated with the laser. Using the pulsed carbon dioxide laser with a flexible waveguide, the laser is adjusted to 250–300 mJ and 8–20 watts. Generally, a layer of fat is left attached to the skin with the dissection plane limited to the loose areolar tissue immediately below the subcutaneous fat. The surgeon applies upward traction to the skin edge, while the assistant applies forward traction ahead of the flap with a gauze sponge and backward traction with a skin hook behind the dissection plane. These maneuvers identify the proper plane of dissection in the loose areolar tissue.

The dissection should proceed smoothly and quickly. A sign that the surgeon is too superficial is if the dissection slows. In this event, the surgeon must usually stop immediately and proceed with the dissection in a deeper plane. For beginners in the use of laser-assisted surgery, it is helpful to undermine the tissues first with a small dissection cannula with saline infusion. The laser may then be used to connect the tunnels that are produced.

4.3.2 Necklift

The surgeon may elect to perform a necklift alone or in conjunction with the cheek or forehead portions of a facelift. While different variations of a corset platysmaplasty have been used by the author in the past, a modification of Giampappa's suture suspension platysmaplasty (1) provides a universal necklift.

Closed liposuction is performed first in a standard fashion. Following this, a 2.5–3.0-cm incision is then made under the chin. The submental skin flap is elevated with the laser (250 mJ, 8–10 watts) between the sternocleidomastoid muscles at a level immediately above the platysma muscle, leaving all the fat on the elevated flap. Little bleeding is seen and minimal ecchymosis is present postoperatively.

The "break" point of the neck is then marked above the hyoid. Slightly above this point, the edges of platysma muscle are grasped and, from the right side, a horizontal mattress suture is placed, suturing the two muscles together but leaving the ends untied. A vertical mattress suture is then placed from the left side, leaving this suture untied also. These sutures, when cinched together, pull the edges of the platysma together and define the muscle edges. If platysma bands are present, a triangle of muscle below the sutures is vaporized with the laser. The use of the laser for the incision and vaporization of muscle is quite bloodless. Monoclear sutures that coapt the lower platysma muscle edges may be used if the bands extend below the thyroid cartilage.

A 2.5–3.0-cm incision is then made in the right postauricular sulcus. This may extend vertically under the auricle to the hairline, if there is significant neck skin excess. The neck skin is then elevated posteriorly to the hairline and anteriorly to connect with the anterior undermining. The laser with a flexible waveguide at 250–300 mJ and 10–15 watts facilitates the bloodless undermining. A short 4-mm endoscope attached to a custom retractor (Karl Storz) enables the emissary veins to be identified and cauterized as needed.

The untied ends of the right platysmaplasty suture are then passed under the skin flap. The posterior edge of platysma is then plicated or imbricated to the mastoid fascia. The platysmaplasty suture is also sutured to the mastoid fascia and tightened. The incisions are then closed.

For the patient with mild to severe neck ptosis who does not require or desire a cheeklift or full facelift, the necklift may be performed alone. For others, it may be performed in conjunction with a cheeklift, an endoscopic forehead lift, or an endoscopic facelift.

4.3.3 Composite Suprafibromuscular Cheeklift with Malar Fat Pad Suspension

While the laser can reduce the swelling and postoperative morbidity seen with standard facelifting (2–4), the most dramatic reduction in these side effects is seen with its use during composite facelifting (5–9). The laser may be used for the dissection "skin to skin."

The incision is made with a 50-mm handpiece (250 mJ, 8–10 watts). The flexible waveguide is then used (250 mJ, 10–20 watts) to dissect the skin flap anteriorly for about 4 cm. Over the malar body, an incision is made through the submucosal aponeurotic system (SMAS) and carried inferiorly. A SMAS flap is elevated over the zygomaticus muscle in a plane above the fibromuscular layer (6). This plane is slightly superficial to the standard composite dissection.

The bloodless field seen during laser dissection demonstrates the fibromuscular SMAS net as a distinct pinkish layer. The loose areolar tissue immediately above this is ideal for laser dissection with the flexible waveguide (250 mJ, 8–10 watts). The dissection is carried past the nasolabial fold.

Dissection must be carried from superior to inferior as the SMAS splits into two leaves. The more superficial leaf of the SMAS runs from superior to inferior. The deeper, inferior leaf of the SMAS passes under the zygomaticus muscle and often the zygomaticus nerve and/or the parotid duct and buccal branch of the facial nerve. In the laser dissection plane above the superior leaf, the facial nerve lies safely below.

The fibromuscular layer is then plicated vertically upward to the malar body, elevating the nasolabial fold and the corner of the mouth. The malar fat pad is also sutured laterosuperiorly to the malar body periosteum. The SMAS flap is then sutured backward to fascia, the skin is trimmed, and the incision is closed.

For a patient who has had a facelift without correction of the nasolabial fold and malar fat pad or for the younger patient with only minimal neck ptosis, the cheeklift may be performed alone. For

48

others, it may be performed in association with the necklift and/or endoscopic forehead lift.

4.3.4 Endoscopic Forehead Lift

While a full discussion of endoscopic face and forehead lifting is beyond the scope of this chapter, it can be said that the laser is an extremely useful instrument for endoscopic facial plastic surgery. Because the endoscopic forehead lift is the most commonly performed endoscopic facial plastic procedure, it will be emphasized here.

The endoscopic forehead lift may be performed in the subcutaneous plane, the subgaleal plane, the subperiosteal plane, or combinations of the three (6–8,10). The laser is most useful for dissections in the subcutaneous and subgaleal planes. To dissect in these planes, the laser is used with the flexible waveguide (250–400 mJ, 10–30 watts). The laser is also useful for incision of the glabellar musculature (corrugator, procerus, and depressor supercilii muscles) and for incision of the arcus marginalis (250 mJ, 8–10 watts).

In the most common endoscopic forehead lift, the laser is used to make five 1.5–2.0-cm incisions (Figure 4.1). Dissection is first performed through the temple incision and then carried medially over the deep temporal fascia. The frontal bone is identified and dissection is performed over it in either the subgaleal or subperiosteal plane to the midline, connecting the temple dissection with the other incisions. If the dissection is performed in the subperiosteal plane, special elevators (Keller–Karl Storz) are used. If the dissection is performed in the subgaleal plane, the laser is used with the waveguide passing through special delivery instruments.

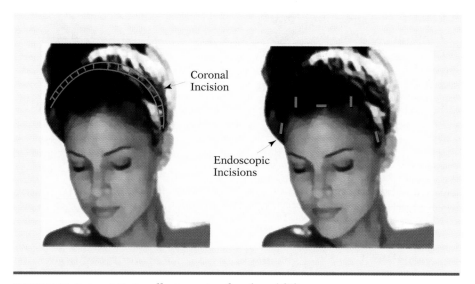

FIGURE 4.1 Minimally invasive forehead lift.

With the endoscope in the central incision and the laser or instrument passed through the midcentral incisions, the dissection is carried downward below the brow. At this point, the periosteum is incised with the laser and the corrugator, procerus, and depressor supercilii are incised. The supraorbital nerve and the supratrochlear nerves are identified and preserved. The laser is most useful for this portion of the procedure. The usual bleeding seen with manual dissection is not encountered, thereby reducing the postoperative morbidity and the need for drains.

The scalp is then undermined posteriorly to the nuchal ridge. Posterior retraction is then used to pull the scalp backward. A screw, k-wire, or suspension suture is used to hold the posterior retraction. The scalp quickly redistributes itself into its new position and the brows are elevated to a predetermined degree.

The endoscopic forehead lift may be performed separately or in conjunction with a necklift or composite facelift. When performed in conjunction with a composite facelift, the dissection is carried down to or over the zygomatic arch.

4.4 SUMMARY

The pulsed carbon dioxide laser with a flexible waveguide is most useful for composite cheeklifting, necklifts, and endoscopic incision and dissection of the forehead and glabellar musculature. While the eventual results of surgery with or without the laser are the same, previous research indicates that the laser diminishes the degree and length of postoperative morbidity seen after rhytidectomy (2–5).

CASE 4.1 MALAR FAT PAD PTOSIS AND JOWLING

A 50-year-old woman complained that she looked old and tired and that her face had fallen, with deeper lines developing between her nose and mouth (Case Figure 4.1A). The patient had had several collagen injections with only transient and marginal results. She had also had two fat injection procedures, which were initially helpful but temporary. The patient did not desire cheek implants because they would make her look like a different person. She just wanted to "look more like (she) used to."

Diagnosis: Malar fat pad ptosis into nasolabial fold and fallen SMAS net with jowl formation.

Procedure: Composite (suprafibromuscular) segmental facelift with SMAS and malar fat pad suspension to the malar body (Case Figures 4.1B, 4.1C).

Postoperative Results: Stabilization of the cheek, jowls, and nasolabial folds (Case Figure 4.1D). Presentable in public with makeup in 12 days. Case Figure 4.1E shows patient–daughter comparison, demonstrating adequate malar fat pad repositioning.

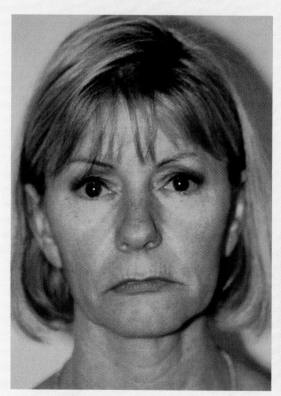

Case 4.1A Before

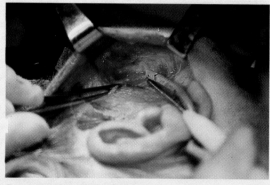

Case 4.1B SMAS flap

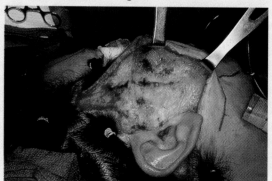

Case 4.1C Malar fat pad suspension

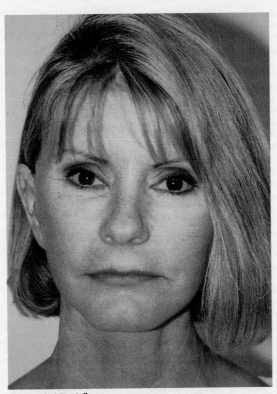

Case 4.1D After

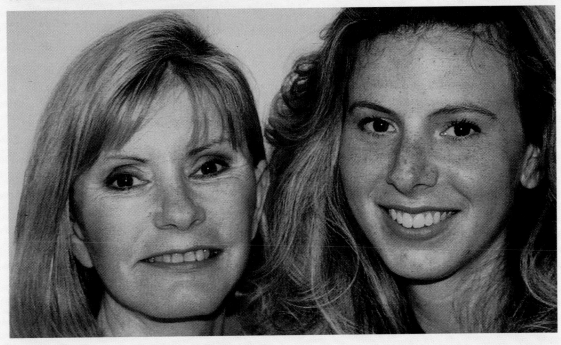

Case 4.1E Patient–daughter comparison.

CASE 4.2 BROW PTOSIS AND FOREHEAD RHYTIDES

A 40-year-old woman complained that she "seemed older and looked like (she) frowned all the time" (Case Figure 4.2A). She had noted these changes in the year prior to presentation and had been raising her brow to compensate for the frowning. She did not desire the forehead lift scars, numbness, and hair thinning that her friend had experienced with surgery.

Diagnosis: Brow ptosis with compensatory forehead rhytides.

Procedure: Laser-assisted endoscopic browlift using the Surgilase XJ carbon dioxide laser. Central frontal elevation in the subgaleal plane with the laser and lateral frontal elevation in the subperiosteal plane. Interruption of the corrugator, procerus, and depressor supercilii muscles with the laser, preserving the supraorbital and supratrochlear nerves (Case Figure 4.2B). Temporal elevation in the deep temporal fascia. Screw fixation of the forehead elevation.

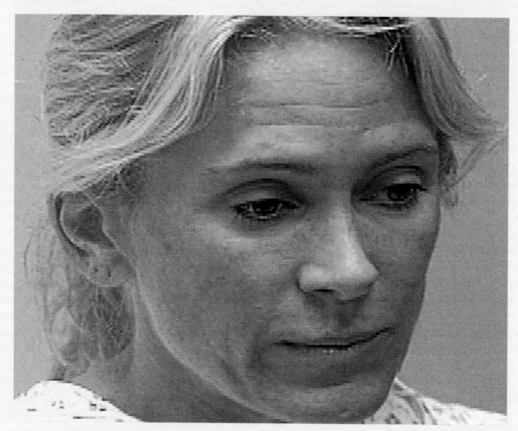

Case 4.2A Before

Postoperative Results: Stable brow elevation and disappearance of rhytides (Case Figure 4.2C). Mild swelling without ecchymosis was experienced. A small area of numbness in the central portion of the forehead remains.

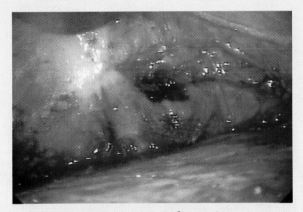

Case 4.2B Intraoperative dissection

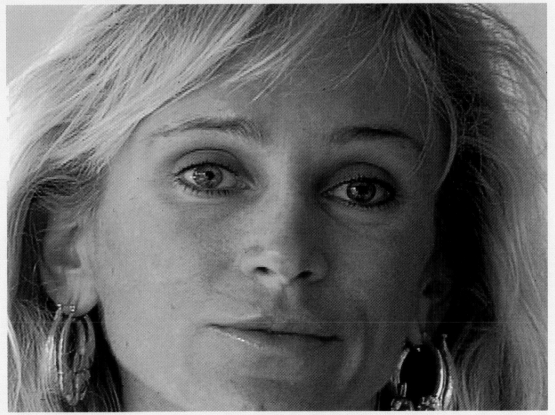

Case 4.2C After

REFERENCES

1. Giampappa VC, DiBernardo A. Suture suspension platysmaplasty. *Am Acad Aesth Restor Surg* 1993 (presentation).
2. Morrow D, Morrow L. Carbon dioxide laser-assisted facelift: a preliminary report. *Am J Cosmetic Surg* 1992;9:159–63.
3. Capriotti RJ. Laser rhytidectomy using the carbon dioxide laser. *Facial Plast Surg Clin North Am* 1993;1:163–72.
4. Apfelberg D. YAG laser meloplasty and blepharoplasty. *Aesth Plast Surg* 1995;19:231–5.
5. Kulich M. Evaluation of the KTP laser in aesthetic facial surgery. *Aesth Plast Surg* (*in press*).
6. Keller GS. Use of the KTP laser in cosmetic surgery. *Am J Cosmetic Surg* 1992;9:177–80.
7. Keller GS. KTP laser rhytidectomy. *Facial Plast Surg Clin North Am* 1993;1:153–62.
8. Keller GS, Cray JC. Rhytidectomy with the Surgilase XJ laser. *Facial Plast Surg Clin North Am* (*in press*).
9. Keller GS. Suprafibromuscular facelifting with periosteal suspension of the SMAS and fat pad of Bichat: tightening the net. *Arch Otolaryngol* (*in press*).
10. Keller GS, Razum NJ, Elliott S, et al. Small incision laser lift for forehead creases and glabellar furrows. *Arch Otolaryngol* 1993;119:632–5.

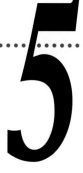

LASER HAIR TRANSPLANTATION

Walter P. Unger, M.D.

5.1 INTRODUCTION

Initially, hair transplantation involved the movement of round pieces of hair-bearing scalp from what was judged to be a permanent donor rim to similar, but somewhat smaller, round sites punched out in the bald or balding recipient area. "Punch transplanting" as this was termed had several significant disadvantages (Table 5.1):

1. If the area being treated still had some hair within it, it would initially be somewhat sparser after transplanting; the punch removed some hair as the recipient area hole was being drilled and the graft that was put in its place lost its hair for a period of 3 months.

2. If the area being treated was completely alopecic, the patient would go through a stage during which he would look somewhat like a "Cupie" doll until dense transplanting had been accomplished. This required at least four operative sessions in most instances.

3. Unless the operator had great skill and experience, even after punch transplanting was completed, the results were unnatural enough that the patient had to make considerable use of careful hairstyling—in particular, concealing the hairline.

Cosmetic Laser Surgery, Edited by Alster, M.D. and Apfelberg, M.D.
ISBN 0471-12242-4   © 1996 Wiley-Liss, Inc.

TABLE 5.1 Advantages and Disadvantages of Hair Transplantation Procedures

PUNCH GRAFTS	TRADITIONAL SLIT GRAFTS	LASER SLIT GRAFTS
• Less even, more unnatural hair growth • More difficult cosmesis between treatment sessions ("Cupie" doll look)	• More natural hairline • "Compression" of grafts • Decreased hair density relative to round grafts • Graft elevation or depression	• More natural distribution of hair • Elimination of compression • No graft elevation or depression • Excellent hemostasis

A solution to the above problems seemed to have been found with the advent of "minigrafting" in which smaller grafts containing only 1–6 hairs were transferred to the recipient area. The smaller grafts could be placed into holes made by an ordinary 16-gauge hypodermic needle (1–2-hair "micrografts"), small round holes made with 1–2-mm diameter punches ("round minigrafts"), or slits made with a scalpel blade ("slit grafts"). Micrografts and slit grafts, in particular, had the advantage of not removing any existing original hair, as the holes or slits could be made between the existing hairs. Because of this, and the cosmetic advantage of a linear rather than round shape, many hair transplant surgeons prefer slit grafts over small, round grafts. Slit grafting, however, has a number of drawbacks of its own:

1. "Compression" of the 1–2-mm wide slit grafts due to their placement within narrow slits made by a scalpel blade. The darker, coarser, more textured, or denser the hair, the more cosmetically unacceptable such compression becomes. The result in such individuals is dark dense lines of coarse hair that are at least as bad-looking as "round grafting in transition," and they are far more difficult to correct.

2. Less hair density than round grafts if one is utilizing comparable amounts of donor tissue. With round grafting, alopecic or potentially alopecic skin is removed, while hair is being added. With scalpel slit grafting, no alopecic or potentially alopecic skin is being eliminated. Thus if one is moving the same amount of donor tissue, the same density cannot be achieved with slit grafts as with round grafts.

3. A tendency to develop graft elevation or depression. Because a 1–2-mm wide graft is being squeezed into a narrow slit, the opportunity for graft elevation or depression increases.

All of the above potential problems with slit grafting are avoided if the slit can be made 1-2 mm wide with, for example, the use of a laser. The problems of compression, decreased hair density, and graft elevation or depression disappear once a 1-2-mm wide recipient site line is produced.

Unfortunately, most carbon dioxide lasers have been associated with unacceptably wide zones of thermal damage adjacent to the lines of incision. It was therefore not until the development of a high-energy, pulsed carbon dioxide laser (Coherent Ultrapulse) that the opportunity to use lasers in hair transplantation became a viable alternative. This particular laser can produce high-energy pulses that are delivered in brief bursts that are shorter than the thermal relaxation time of skin [695 milliseconds (ms)]. Photomicrographs of incisions deep enough to receive slit grafts revealed zones of thermal damage that were only 20–50 micrometers (μm) wide at the level of the hair matrix (Figure 5.1), thus sparing adjacent hair follicles.

5.2 BACKGROUND

An initial study on the use of the high-energy, pulsed carbon dioxide (Ultrapulse) laser in hair transplantation consisted of hair counts in grafts transplanted into laser-prepared and scalpel-prepared sites in similar but contralateral locations in the recipient area of ten patients. After 4 months, hair survival in the grafts placed into laser-

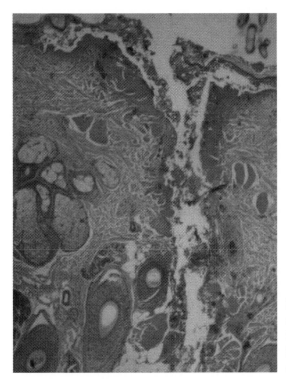

FIGURE 5.1 A photomicrograph of a laser-produced "slit." The purple color reflects significant thermal damage. At the level of the hair matrices, it is 20–50 μm wide and completely spares adjacent hair follicles.

prepared slit sites was greater than for those placed into scalpel-prepared slit sites in four out of ten patients, equal in five patients, and less in one patient. In addition, hair growth occurred earlier (7.5–9.0 weeks) in laser site grafts in five of the ten patients. The results of this study were reported in 1994 (1). Prior to that publication, however, an increasing number of grafts had been placed into laser-prepared slit sites, each time waiting to see that satisfactory hair growth occurred in the previous smaller number of test grafts. Figure 5.2 demonstrates the results seen in a patient in whom 85 grafts were placed into scalpel-prepared slit sites on the left side of an alopecic area and 85 grafts were placed in laser-prepared slit sites on the right side of the same area.

The most promising finding has been a more "even" and therefore more natural appearing distribution of hair over the laser-treated areas without the slightest "compression." Furthermore, bald or potentially bald skin is ablated by the laser so that the second most important disadvantage of slit grafting—decreased density with the same amount of transplanted hair—is also eliminated. Third, the amount of bleeding in the recipient area can be almost completely controlled by adjusting the energy density (millijoules) of the laser. Although one can operate in a virtually dry or bloodless field, all bleeding should *not* be eliminated. A little bleeding assures that the grafts will get adequate and quick revascularization and nutrition. The blood may also act as a "biologic glue." In two early treatment patients in whom all bleeding had been eliminated, one or two grafts fell out several days postoperatively because there wasn't enough bleeding to fix them in place (1).

5.3 LASER HAIR TRANSPLANTATION TECHNIQUE

5.3.1 Patient and Donor Site Selection

Patient selection is similar to that for all types of hair transplantation and has been described in great detail elsewhere (2). In general, one assesses the long-term donor to recipient area ratio in order to establish how much of the bald, or potentially bald, area one can reasonably hope to cover with transplanted grafts. The hairline is begun and ended where one expects the ultimate anteriormost/supe-

(Facing page)

FIGURE 5.2 (a) Eighty-five slit sites to the right side of the midsclap, 1 week after treatment. (b) Laser-treated area 5 months after treatment. Note the diffuse nature of hair growing in this area. (c) Another view of the laser-treated area on the right side of the midscalp. The comparable area on the left side was treated with scalpel slits. Hair growth in this latter area is not as diffuse and looks somewhat "compressed" when compared to the right side.

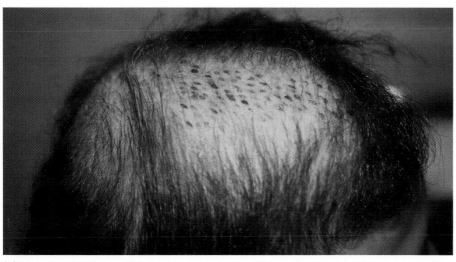

(a)

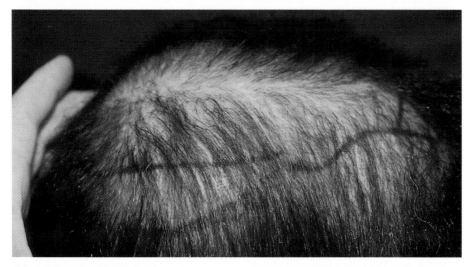

(b)

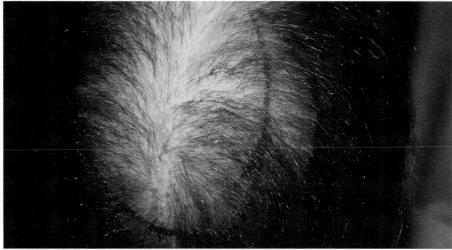

(c)

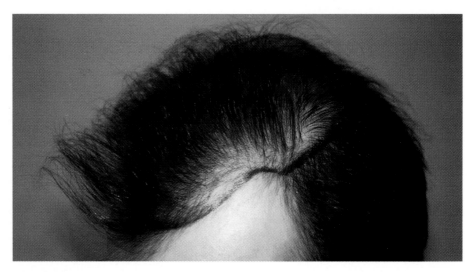

FIGURE 5.3   The black crayon denotes the borders of the area to be treated. Note the area immediately superior to the crayon line in the temporal area. This site still has a reasonable hair density, but wetting it reveals the thinning process has already begun there. By transplanting through this still hair-bearing area at the same time as more obviously sparse areas are being transplanted, the patient/doctor will minimize the chance of having to "chase" an enlarging bald area.

riormost points of the temporal hair will be, and its midline point is chosen so that the hairline, when viewed laterally, runs more or less parallel to the ground. An effort is made to transplant throughout residual hair-bearing areas that can reasonably be expected to eventually become alopecic, thus minimizing the chance of having to "chase" an enlarging bald area (Figure 5.3).

The factors affecting the shape and size of the permanently hair-bearing "donor area" have also been reviewed extensively (3). A "safe" donor area for 80% of patients under the age of 80 years has been suggested by a study in which hair density in the persistent rim was recorded in 322 men ranging from 65 to 79 years of age (Figure 5.4).

5.3.2 Anesthesia

The donor site is anesthesized with a tumescent anesthetic solution prepared by adding 4.8 ml of 2% lidocaine without epinephrine, 0.52 ml of $NaHCO_3$ (1 mEq/ml), and 0.40 ml of fresh epinephrine (1:1000) to a 100-ml bag of normal saline. Up to 100 cc are infiltrated slowly into the areas to be harvested, through a single injection site, using a $18 \times 3\frac{1}{2}$ inch spinal needle (4). The recipient area is anesthetized utilizing a field block prepared with 2% lidocaine with 1:100,000 epinephrine and 50 mEq/liter of sodium bicarbonate—the latter added to minimize the pain of injection (5). A 2% solution

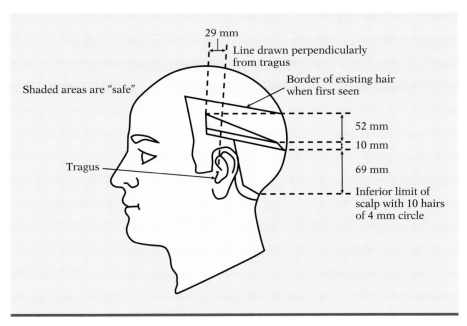

FIGURE 5.4 The above "safe" donor area, for 80% of men under the age of 80 years, was derived from an objective study of the permanent rim hair density in 322 men aged 65–79 years. (From ref. 6, with permission.)

of lidocaine with 1:100,000 epinephrine (but no sodium bicarbonate) is used to produce a second field block superior to the first, and even more superiorly, a solution of 1:200,000 epinephrine is employed. Tumescent anesthesia is not used by the author in the recipient area because of the production of additional postoperative edema and the difficulty of estimating accurate spacing of grafts once the distention caused by the tumescent anesthesia has resolved. Regional nerve blocks are utilized only for patients in whom it is more difficult than average to obtain complete anesthesia using the tumescent technique described earlier.

5.3.3 Donor Area Harvesting

The donor tissue is obtained by using a triple- or quadruple-bladed knife to excise strips of skin, each of which is 2.5–3.0 mm wide. After cautery of bleeding vessels, the wound is normally closed in a single layer using a simple running stitch and 2-0 Supramid on a CL20 needle. The strips will carefully be cut into sections containing 1–6 hairs each. Graft tissue is obtained from the inferior occipital area, the superior occipital area, and occasionally the temporal area. Each area produces grafts with varying hair density, texture, and possibly color. This provides the operator with more flexibility in producing a good aesthetic result by using grafts with the most advantageous characteristics for specific areas in the recipient site

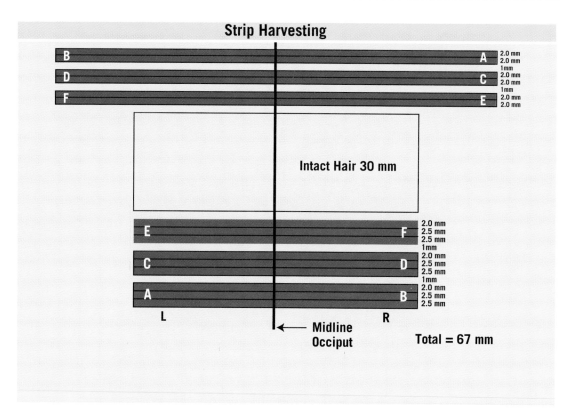

FIGURE 5.5 The donor area shown will produce, in most patients, six sessions (A-E) of slit grafts 350–400 and 100–125 micrografts per session. The inact hair zone may also be deleted if there is any concern that there will not be 67 mm of good donor area thus reducing the required donor area to one that is only 37 mm high.

(6). Fine hairs in the inferior occipital area and temporal area, for example, are ideal for producing natural-looking hairlines. Coarse and/or denser hair from the superior occipital area is more suitable for producing greater density more posteriorly in the recipient area. Figure 5.5 demonstrates the approach taken for obtaining donor tissue for subsequent sessions. Each time a new donor strip is harvested, the old adjacent scar is excised with it, so that ultimately only two narrow donor site scars will persist in the parieto-occipital area, and one in each of the temporal areas. In most patients, it is not difficult to obtain enough donor material from the parieto-occipital area for six or more sessions, each of which will consist of approximately 350–400 slit grafts and 100–125 micrografts.

5.3.4 Recipient Area Preparation and Hair Placement

Although grafts must appear to be distributed in a relatively random way in the recipient area in order to produce a natural-looking result, the organization of grafts in the area must be anything other than random if an even distribution of hair is to be achieved. In brief, a very highly "organized disorganization" is utilized (7). The author recommends the following four parameters: grafts in session one should be (a) 3 mm apart and (b) consistently 1 mm anterior or posterior to their neighbor. In addition, (c) the angle of incision should be approximately 45° and (d) the direction of incision should follow the direction of the original hair in that area. During session two, the slits will be made midway between those of the first session. Conventional slit grafting is currently used in session three to fill the remaining spaces (Figure 5.6). Acquiring the skill to accurately and consistently accomplish these goals takes time and experience and is a major component of learning the "art" of hair transplantation. Usually, three sessions of slit grafting will produce excellent cosmetic results. If hair characteristics are particularly good—for example, fine, dense, and light-colored—even one or two sessions may produce a very satisfactory result. One of the distinct advantages of the

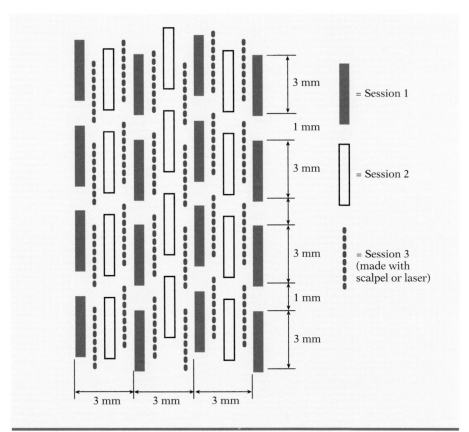

FIGURE 5.6   Spacing of laser slits. A laser "slit" produced with a 0.2-mm spot in focus results in a wound that gapes to approximately 0.5 mm. The distance between adjacent slits made during the same session is 3 mm. This would allow complete filling of the site in three sessions if that were the objective. For the present, scalpel slits are used for the third session (a) to provide a "margin of safety," protecting adjacent transplanted hair from possible laser thermal damage ("margin of safety" is probably not necessary) and (b) because complete filling in some areas, such as the hairline zone, is often not the objective.

64

laser for hair transplanting is that it lends itself to the addition of a computer-driven "scanner" that can move the laser beam in a very accurate and consistent fashion. Such a scanner is currently under development and will be available in the near future.

The most common settings for the laser utilizing a 0.2-mm focused spot is 12–15 watts and 300–350 millijoules (mJ). The settings are adjusted to produce an incision that is neither too deep nor too shallow by changing the power (watts), and to produce a small amount of bleeding by adjusting the energy (millijoules). The spot is moved along at a speed such that a 3 mm long line is produced in 0.8–0.99 seconds. Moving the light more slowly results in additional charring and deeper penetration than is advisable or necessary. Moving it more quickly results in insufficient penetration. Exposure time is therefore limited to 0.8–0.9 seconds in order to "discipline" the operator to move the beam at the appropriate speed. A computer-driven scanner will thus provide an ideal and consistent rate of movement, as well as proper spacing and positioning of grafts.

5.3.5 Graft Insertion and Bandaging

The previously prepared grafts are inserted into the laser sites with their hair directed parallel to the original hair in the area. Care is taken that no hair is accidentally trapped under a graft and that the grafts are positioned flush with the surrounding skin. Bacitracin ointment is used in both the recipient area and the donor area. Telfa is placed over the recipient area and an overnight pressure bandage is applied. The bandage is removed the next day and the area is cleansed with hydrogen peroxide. The patient's hair can be carefully washed, dried, and styled by a medical assistant or nurse in those offices equipped to do so on the morning after surgery.

5.3.6 Postoperative Course

Patients are instructed to apply bacitracin ointment three or more times per day to the grafts as well as to the donor area for the following week. This is an important step in that a small amount of superficial deepithelialization is present around each laser site. This leaves the recipient area susceptible to infection, which could impair hair survival. It also minimizes the production of crust over the grafts. Sutures are removed from the donor area in 7–10 days. With large numbers of grafts (75 or more), hair regrowth usually occurs 2–6 weeks later than that normally seen with conventional slit grafting. The routine use of 3% minoxidil solution twice daily for the first 5 weeks postoperatively may help in minimizing this possibility.

A variable amount of postoperative edema and crusting occur but usually resolve completely within 10–14 days. Postoperative pain is usually minimal; however, patients are given acetaminophen with 60 mg codeine (Tylenol #3), oxycodone (Percocet), and meperidine hydrochloride (Demerol) to take as required. Few, however, require anything more than Tylenol #3.

All of the complications that may occur with standard transplantation may occur with laser transplantation (8). As indicated earlier, there is a slightly increased propensity to develop infection due to laser-induced deepithelialization of adjacent skin, but this risk is markedly reduced with the diligent use of antibiotic ointment postoperatively.

5.4 RESULTS OF LASER SLIT TRANSPLANTATION

Given similar hair characteristics, hair distribution is significantly more "even" and natural-looking than that observed with either slit grafting or round minigrafting, yet hair density is comparable to round grafting. The hair is so evenly distributed that sometimes it appears as if no transplantation has occurred, even after only one session (see Figure 5.2). The less ideal the hair characteristics, the more strikingly advantageous the laser becomes. Conversely, the better the hair characteristics, the less advantage one gains with the laser. In brief, the laser appears to combine the best aspects of round grafting and slit grafting, while at the same time eliminating their most important disadvantages.

While only slit grafting with lasers has been investigated thus far, there is no reason that any principles that apply to laser slit grafting cannot be applied in the use of lasers to make round, square, or hexagonal recipient sites of varying sizes, if these are preferred. Variations in approaches may also be introduced to minimize potential problems and/or maximize results. For example, the Ultrapulse laser is currently being used to produce 2-mm round recipient holes that only penetrate as far as the mid-dermis so that dilators can then be used to extend the holes deep enough for acceptance of grafts (J. Fulton, *personal communication*). Because deeper vessels are spared any potential laser damage, entire recipient areas may be treated at once. Reports of less postoperative edema and pain than usually found with conventional hair transplantation have been encouraging. Still other techniques are being investigated and the future holds much promise for even faster and more effective laser-assisted hair transplantation procedures.

5.5 SUMMARY

We are on the threshold of a new phase in hair transplantation: laser hair transplanting. Results are encouraging and sometimes impressively superior to that seen with conventional transplantation techniques. On the other hand, the exact role that laser transplanting will play in this area of cosmetic surgery remains to be determined. It appears that it will be most advantageous for the treatment of patients with less ideal hair characteristics for traditional transplantation and for novice transplant surgeons. It may, however, offer advantages that will appeal to a far larger group of patients and surgeons as a result of its superior hemostatic properties and ease of application.

REFERENCES

1. Unger W, David L. Laser hair transplantation. *J Dermatol Surg Oncol* 1994;20:515–21.
2. Unger W. Planning. In: Unger W, ed. *Hair transplantation*, 3rd ed. New York: Marcel Dekker, 1995;105–58.
3. Unger W. Delineating the "safe" donor area in hair transplanting. *J Am Acad Cosmetic Surg* 1994;4:239–43.
4. Coleman W III, Klein JA. Use of the tumescent technique for scalp surgery, dermabrasion, and soft tissue reconstruction *J. Dermatol Surg Oncol* 1992;18:130–5.
5. Unger W. Anesthesia. In: Unger W, ed. *Hair transplantation*, 3rd ed. New York: Marcel Dekker, 1995;165–81.
6. Unger W. The donor site. In: Unger W, ed. *Hair transplantation*, 3rd ed. New York: Marcel Dekker, 1995;182–214.
7. Unger W. The recipient area. In: Unger W, ed. *Hair transplantation*, 3rd ed. New York: Marcel Dekker, 1995;215–321.
8. Unger W. Complications. In: Unger W, ed. *Hair transplantation*, 3rd ed. New York: Marcel Dekker, 1995;363–74.

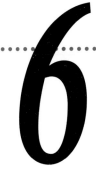

LASER-ASSISTED UVULOPALATOPLASTY FOR SNORING

Yosef P. Krespi, M.D.

Maurice M. Khosh, M.D.

6.1 INTRODUCTION

Snoring has long been described as a socially disturbing factor. Only relatively recently have the adverse medical effects of snoring, and its association with obstructive sleep apnea (OSA) and upper airway resistance syndrome (UARS), been recognized. It is now accepted that snoring, upper airway resistance syndrome, and obstructive sleep apnea describe a continuum of sleep disturbance with progressively greater health hazards.

Various methods have been utilized to alleviate snoring and/or OSA. They include behavior modification, sleep positioning, continuous airway pressure, and uvulopalatopharyngoplasty as described by Ikematsu (1). Laser technology has been applied to the treatment of snoring in the form of laser-assisted uvulopalatoplasty (LAUP). LAUP allows treatment of snoring and mild OSA in an ambulatory setting with local anesthesia. The result has been reduced surgical morbidity and health care cost.

6.2 SLEEP DISTURBANCE

6.2.1 Snoring

Snoring is a loud and recurrent breath sound, with variable intensity and frequency, that occurs upon inspiration during sleep. It is generated by the vibration of the soft tissue structures in the pharynx.

Cosmetic Laser Surgery, Edited by Alster, M.D. and Apfelberg, M.D.
ISBN 0471-12242-4   © 1996 Wiley-Liss, Inc.

Epidemiological studies indicate that snoring is common in the general population. Lugaresi (2) in a study of 5713 individuals showed that 19% of adults describe themselves as habitual snorers. This corresponds to 24% of the male and 15% of the female population.

Snoring has long been ignored by most of the medical community and addressed as a purely social problem, with detrimental effects on relationships with bed partners, roommates, or housemates. Sleep specialists have proposed a classification system for snoring intensity: *grade I:* occasional snoring, usually while the sleeper is lying on his/her back, is overtired, or has drunk too much alcohol and eaten too much food; *grade II:* very loud, frequent snoring that occurs in all body positions, continues throughout the night, and can be heard from a room away; *grade III:* extremely loud snoring that can be heard throughout the entire house, commonly associated with obstructive sleep apnea (3). Chronic snorers often report restless sleep, morning headaches, and fatigue. They may demonstrate daytime listlessness and hypersomnolence.

6.2.2 Upper Airway Resistance Syndrome

Upper airway resistance syndrome (UARS) is described as chronic daytime sleepiness, habitual snoring (grade II or III), and sleep fragmentation. In UARS no significant apneic pauses or oxygen desaturation is manifest in sleep studies; however, daytime nap studies are frequently positive. UARS may be a risk factor for hypertension, angina pectoris, cerebral infarction, pulmonary hypertension, and congestive heart failure (4–6), conditions more commonly associated with OSA (6).

6.2.3 Obstructive Sleep Apnea

Obstructive sleep apnea (OSA) is the most severe end of the sleep disturbance continuum. It is characterized by periodic apneas and hypopneas that produce asphyxia and arousal from sleep. The disease entity was first described by Guilleminault et al. (7) in 1976. Diagnosis of OSA is confirmed by polysomnography. Several levels of polysomnography are available; however, level I overnight polysomnography is considered the most reliable (8). In level I overnight polysomnography, the patient is monitored by pulse oximetry, electroencephalography (EFG), electroculography (EOG), electrocardiography (ECG), nasal and oral airflow measurements, submental and anterior tibial electromyography (EMG), plethysmography, sleep position, and manometry (9) in the presence of an attendant.

OSA can be classified according to the Apnea–Hypopnea Index (AHI) and oxygen desaturation. The AHI or the Respiratory Disturbance Index is the number of apneic and hypopneic episodes per hour of sleep. Obstructive sleep apnea is considered mild if the AHI is between 5 and 20, moderate if the AHI is between 30 and 40, and severe if the AHI is greater than 40. The incidence of OSA may be as high as 4% in the general population and 5–10% in adult men (10,11). As previously mentioned, OSA has been associated with cardiac, pulmonary, and cerebrovascular problems (6,12).

6.3 DIAGNOSIS

Diagnosis of snoring is made primarily by history, much of which can be obtained from the patient's bed partner. The character and consistency of the snoring are examined to determine its severity and possible presence of OSA. Frequent episodes of breathing cessation followed by sudden and intensified snoring is a strong indication of OSA. A detailed survey that explores the snorer's medical condition, sleeping position, alcohol and sedative intake, and weight changes is an important part of the history.

Physical examination should include complete evaluation of the nose, nasopharynx, oral cavity, oropharynx, hypopharynx, and larynx. Flexible fiber optic nasolaryngoscopy aids this examination as well as allowing the performance of a Müeller maneuver. The Müeller maneuver consists of inhaling against a closed mouth and nose to create maximal negative pressure in the upper airway. This aids in the detection of any collapsing site in the pharynx (13). Polysomnography is indicated if the suspicion of OSA exists. Diagnostic modalities such as computed tomography (CT) scanning, magnetic resonance imaging (MRI), cephalometric analysis, manometry, and acoustic reflection analysis have been described as tools in determining the sight of obstruction in OSA (14–19).

6.4 PATHOPHYSIOLOGY

Snoring originates from vibration of the soft tissue structures in the pharynx, including the soft palate, uvula, tonsils, tonsillar pillars, tongue base, and the posterior and lateral walls of the pharynx. These vibrations occur because of airflow turbulence in the sleeper's pharynx, originating either in the nose (i.e., due to turbinate enlargement or septal deviation) or in the oropharynx. The turbulent airflow produces a flutter-valve effect in the collapsible pharyngeal tissues, which can be likened to a flag snapping back and forth in a stiff breeze.

OSA results from the collapse of the pharyngeal walls in response to negative inspiratory pressure in the upper airway. Pharyngeal musculature hypotonicity allows upper airway collapse at more modest negative inspiratory pressures. Narrowing of the upper airway, due to any reason, increases the velocity of airflow via the Bernoulli effect and reduces the intraluminal pressure. This facilitates pharyngeal collapse or soft tissue flutter, leading to apnea or snoring.

6.5 RISK FACTORS FOR SNORING AND OSA

6.5.1 Obesity

Obesity represents the most common risk factor for snoring and OSA. Keidar et al. (20), in a review of 124 individuals with snoring and a level I polysomnography, found that over 80% of the patients were obese (Body Mass Index greater than 27) and that obesity showed a strong correlation with the severity of OSA. Possible mechanisms by which obesity causes or aggravates snoring include physical narrowing of the pharynx due to bulk, fat infiltration of pharyngeal muscle fibers (21), and poor pharyngeal muscle tone.

6.5.2 Muscular Laxity

Issa and Sullivan (22) have shown that snorers tend to have pharyngeal collapse at more moderate negative pharyngeal pressure, a finding indicative of absence or insufficiency of pharyngeal dilator muscles' response to hypoxia.

Most snoring occurs during rapid eye movement (REM) sleep. This corresponds to periods of maximal muscle relaxation, especially in the neck. Lying in the supine position aggravates snoring because the relaxed tongue tends to fall posteriorly into the airway due to gravity.

6.5.3 Drugs and Smoking

Ingestion of tranquilizers, antihistamines, or alcohol prior to sleep can aggravate snoring by causing excessive flaccidity of the upper airway. Alcohol induces vasodilation and edema of the pharyngeal mucosa, while depressing the central respiratory centers centrally and selectively increasing the hypotonia of the pharyngeal dilating muscle (23).

Smoking may exacerbate snoring by increasing upper airway resistance secondary to changes in mucociliary clearance (24), increased production of mucus, and irritation and swelling of the mucous membranes.

6.6 HORMONAL AND CONGENITAL ABNORMALITIES

Hypothyroidism can induce myxedematous changes and altered muscular contractile properties, as well as macroglossia, pharnygeal mucosal thickening, and facial skeletal changes (25). The above noted effects can induce or exacerbate snoring and OSA.

Congenital craniofacial abnormalities can contribute to upper airway obstruction in the form of micrognathia, maxillary hypoplasia, choanal atresia, decreased pharyngeal circumference, distorted pharyngeal orientation, hypotonia of pharyngeal musculature, macroglossia, and laryngeal or tracheal anomalies (26).

6.7 MANAGEMENT MODALITIES

6.7.1 Nonsurgical Management

Surgical procedures to address snoring entail certain risks and discomfort. It is therefore prudent to attempt medical intervention or behavioral modification in appropriate circumstances. Weight reduction, elimination of tranquilizers, avoidance of alcohol prior to sleep, and smoking cessation are important steps in initial management of snoring and obstructive sleep apnea. Treatment of nasal allergies, when present, and thyroid supplementation in hypothyroid patients is indicated.

In grade I snoring, sleep positioning or application of nasal stents may be sufficient. In patients with OSA, continuous positive airway pressure (CPAP) represents the optimal medical management. The CPAP machine is adjusted to overcome the negative pressure in the upper airway during sleep. CPAP thereby prevents pharyngeal collapse and airway obstruction.

Since both medical and behavioral management require prolonged follow-up and/or adherence to a restrictive life-style, not all patients are able to comply. Additionally, many patients do not respond to conservative treatment measures. Surgical management is generally preferred by younger, middle-aged individuals.

6.7.2 Surgical Options

Nasal surgery including septoplasty, turbinectomy, or repair of alar collapse may be necessary in patients with nasal airway obstruction. The surgical treatment of choice for snoring, prior to the introduction of LAUP, was uvulopalatopharyngoplasty (UPPP) (27–29). UPPP was first introduced by Ikematsu (1) in 1964 as a surgical treatment of snoring. In 1981, UPPP was utilized to treat obstructive sleep apnea by Fujita (3). Potential disadvantages of UPPP include the need for general anesthesia and severe postoperative pain. UPPP may be complicated by temporary or permanent velopharyngeal insufficiency, voice changes, and foreign body sensation in the pharynx. The latter may be attributed to loss of the uvula, which acts as a drip spout for pharyngeal mucus and sweeps the posterior pharyngeal wall clear of secretions (30).

LAUP is a technique developed by Kamami in France in the late 1980s (27). It was introduced in the United States as a treatment for snoring without apnea in 1992. The procedure is designed to correct airway obstruction and soft tissue vibration at the level of the soft palate, by reducing and stiffening the tissues in the velum and the uvula.

72 6.8 LASER-ASSISTED UVULOPALATOPLASTY (LAUP)

6.8.1 Contraindications

Absolute contraindications to LAUP in an office setting are relatively few. They include significant sleep apnea (AHI greater than 30), uncontrolled hypertension, trismus, cleft palate, preexisting velopharyngeal insufficiency, uncooperative patients, and anatomical source of snoring other than the oropharynx.

Caution should be exercised in patients who use their voice professionally or play wind instruments. Linguistic constraints for certain languages that use the soft palate or the uvula extensively, such as Arabic, Russian, Hebrew, and Farsi, may also be a consideration. Patients with allergies to local anesthetics and a hyperactive gag reflex should be treated under general anesthesia.

6.8.2 Procedure

LAUP is performed in an upright sitting position in an otolaryngology examination chair. A topical anesthetic such as benzocaine 20% is sprayed in the posterior oral cavity over the soft palate, tonsils, and uvula. After 3 minutes, a mixture of 1.0 cc of 2% lidocaine with 1:100,000 epinephrine and 0.5 cc of 0.5% bupivacaine is injected into the junction of the soft palate and the uvula bilaterally and into the base of the uvula. If laser ablation of the tonsils and the tonsillar pillars is to be performed, injection is also given into the superior junction of the anterior and posterior pillars bilaterally.

Surgical utilization of the laser is commenced after allowing 10 minutes for the anesthetic to take effect and for vasoconstriction to occur. A carbon dioxide laser is preferred due to its wide availability and ease of use. The carbon dioxide laser provides adequate coagulation for the diameter of vessels encountered in this procedure. The following explanation outlines LAUP performance with the carbon dioxide laser.

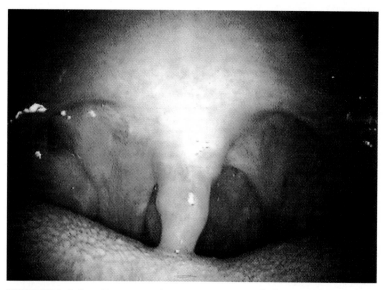

FIGURE 6.1 Preoperative appearance of the oropharynx.

The patient and staff are equipped with protective goggles, and conventional laser safety rules are followed. Power is set at 18–20 watts in the continuous mode. The tongue is retracted inferiorly with an ebonized tongue depressor, which has an integrated smoke evacuation channel. Through and through, full thickness, vertical trenches measuring 1.0–1.5 cm are fashioned on the free edge of the soft palate at either side of the uvula. These trenches are created using a focused beam and a special handpiece with a backstop. The patient is asked to inhale, and the laser is activated during slow exhalation in order to avoid inhalation of the plume.

Shortening and thinning of the uvula are carried out with the regular carbon dioxide laser handpiece in the defocused mode or with the Swiftlase (Sharplan Laser, Inc., Allendale, NJ) flash scanner (28,29). The uvula is reduced to 70–80% of its original dimension by coring it in a cephalic direction (Figures 6.1 and 6.2). Overall, the goal is to reduce the length and reshape the soft palate and uvula. Care must be taken not to burn the mucosal covering of the soft palate and the uvula excessively. The uvula is shortened by ablating the muscle from within, creating a "fish-mouth" appearance, while preserving the mucosa of the base of the uvula on the nasal and oral surfaces. Light bleeding during surgery can occur in 3% of patients (28,29). Bleeding is easily controlled by applying silver nitrate. OSA patients with enlarged tonsils and redundant pharyngeal folds can be helped by the reduction of the upper portion of the pharyngeal folds and tonsils utilizing the Swiftlase system.

Immediately following the procedure, the patient gargles with a cold water and hydrogen peroxide mixture. Typically, LAUP requires two to four treatments spaced a minimum of 1 month apart (31).

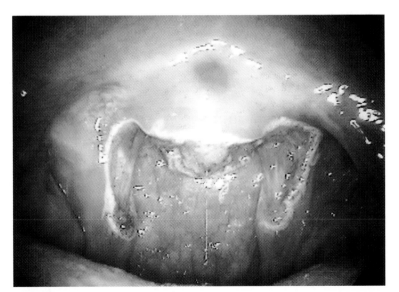

FIGURE 6.2 Immediate postoperative appearance of the oropharynx. Note the char-free ablation of the uvula and lateral palatal folds which result following Swiftlase flash scanner CO_2 laser treatment.

74

Elapsed time between the procedures allows proper healing of the soft palate mucosa. The endpoint of LAUP is determined when significant reduction or complete elimination of snoring has occurred. Confirmation is obtained by patient or partner history and/or by the inability of the patient to perform voluntary "snoring" (28).

Ellis et al. (32) have described a modification of LAUP as described above. They propose using the Nd:YAG contact laser at a power setting of 10 watts to remove a central longitudinal strip of mucosa from the surface of the soft palate. The mucosal ablation is 1.5 cm wide and extends from the junction of the soft and hard palate to the uvula. They explain that allowing the mucosa to heal by secondary intention results in stiffening of the soft palate. This stiffening causes reduction of palatal flutter and, hence, diminution of snoring.

6.8.3 Efficacy

Krespi et al. (28) reviewed 280 patients who underwent LAUP in the office, with a 3-month to 2-year follow-up. They reported 84% elimination of snoring and an additional 7% reduction of snoring. Carenfelt (33) reported 85% total or near total elimination of snoring during a short-term follow-up (duration not specified) of 60 patients. Kamami (27) in a review of 31 patients with a maximal follow-up of 18 months reported 77% elimination or significant reduction of snoring. Ellis et al. (32) published the results of laser palatoplasty in 16 patients with 3–6-month follow-up. The surgical technique described by Ellis et al. was slightly different, in that only a central longitudinal strip of mucosa was removed from the surface of the soft palate. This resulted in 85% elimination or significant reduction of snoring.

Long-term results of LAUP treatment for snoring are not yet available due to the novelty of the procedure. It is possible that prolonged follow-up will reveal more modest success for this operation. Sequert et al. (34) reported on 70 patients who underwent LAUP, as compared to 63 patients who had classical uvulopalatoplasty. The results were rated satisfactory by 54% of the carbon dioxide laser-treated patients as compared to 78% for classical surgery.

6.8.4 Postoperative Instructions

Patients may resume regular activities immediately following surgery. A soft, bland diet with avoidance of citrus products is recommended. Aggressive hydration, humidification, and steam inhalation are emphasized. Mucous membrane dehydration is thought to be an important source of postoperative pain. Viscous xylocaine is used to relieve pain every 4 hours as needed. Gargling with diluted hydrogen peroxide or nonalcoholic mouthwashes is recommended. The need for analgesics varies according to each patient's tolerance. Various analgesics from acetaminophen, to acetaminophen with codeine, to oxycodone hydrochloride can be used. Prophylactic antibiotics are prescribed for every patient. Steroids, however, are not indicated.

6.8.5 Complications

Reported complications for LAUP are rare. Moderate to severe pain is the major side effect of the procedure. Pain intensity reaches its peak 4–5 days postoperatively, with complete relief of symptoms in 2 weeks. Pain is usually well controlled with hydration, anesthetic gel, and oral analgesics. Most patients report some degree of weight loss, typically less than 10 pounds over the course of treatment. Healing occurs by formation of eschar in 3–5 days following the procedure. Complete mucosal healing takes place following the slough of eschar in about 12 days.

Intraoperative bleeding can occur in 3% of the patients. Bleeding is usually from the apex of the palate trench incision and is stopped with application of silver nitrate. No patients have required hosptial admission or transfusion (27–29,33,35). Krespi et al. (28) reported two vasovagal episodes following injection of the local anesthetic in a review of 280 patients. Only one episode of delayed bleeding has been encountered in more than 2000 LAUP treatments.

Velopharyngeal insufficiency, either temporary or permanent, has not been reported, probably due to the graded surgical approach. Nasopharyngeal stenosis has not been encountered. In order to avoid this complication, it is important to use a special laser hand-piece with a backstop to make the palatal incisions. The nasopharyngeal mucosa is thus protected from injury and synechia formation between the velum and the nasopharynx is prevented.

Approximately 40% of patients may complain of "scratchy" or "dry mucous" sensation in the throat. This is usually self-limited and resolves within 2 months.

6.9 SUMMARY

Laser-assisted uvuloplasty (LAUP) is an effective method for treating patients with loud, habitual snoring, upper airway resistance syndrome, and mild obstructive sleep apnea. LAUP offers several advantages to the classical uvulopalatopharyngoplasty, including reduced cost, decreased operative morbidity, diminished postoperative pain, and abbreviated convalescence period, as well as avoidance of general anesthesia.

LAUP as an office procedure performed under local anesthesia has proved to be a safe and effective method of alleviating bothersome snoring. The surgery is undertaken in stages to allow "titration" of tissue removal with minimal risk of overcorrection. Patient selection requires a careful review of the medical history and a thorough physical evaluation. The nose, tongue base, and hypopharynx should be ruled out as the primary site of airway obstruction. Polysomnography is indicated in those patients at risk for OSA. LAUP, when performed in properly selected candidates, can result in excellent clinical outcome and patient satisfaction.

CASE 6.1 THICKENED UVULA RESULTING IN SNORING

A 45-year-old man was seen for evaluation of snoring. His wife had refused to sleep in the same bedroom for the previous 3 years due to the intensity of his snoring. His wife denied episodes of breathing cessation. The patient did not smoke or consume alcohol or sedatives.

Examination: Mild obesity at 5 feet 8 inches height and 179 lb weight (calculated Body Mass Index = 27.4). Mild hypertension was present. Nasal examination did not demonstrate significant septal deviation or turbinate enlargement. Intraoral evaluation revealed a flattened palate, elongated thick uvula, and redundant lateral pharyngeal folds. Fiber optic nasopharyngoscopy showed nonenlarged lingual tonsils and absence of hypopharyngeal collapse on Müller maneuver. (Case Figure 6.1A shows baseline appearance of oropharynx.)

Diagnosis: Snoring due to obesity, thickened uvula, and redundant lateral pharyngeal folds.

Anesthesia: Topical benzocaine 20% spray applied to the posterior oral cavity, followed by injection of a mixture of 1.0 cc of 2% lidocaine with 1:100,000 epinephrine and 0.5 cc of 0.5% bupivicaine into soft palate.

Procedure: Two laser-assisted uvulopalatoplasty (LAUP) procedures at 6 week intervals were performed using the carbon dioxide laser at 18-watts continuous mode. Full thickness vertical trenches measuring 1.0 cm were made on either side of the uvula with a focused beam. Thinning out of the uvula was performed with the Swiftlase flash scanner to reduce the uvula's size by 70–80%. (Case Figure 6.1B shows the oropharynx immediately after the first LAUP treatment.)

Postoperative Results: The patient's snoring is now nearly inaudible and he is unable to perform a voluntary snort. (Case Figure 6.1C shows the appearance of the oropharynx 2 months after completion of the second LAUP procedure.) The patient and his wife are again able to share a bed. The patient reports better quality of sleep, ability to dream, and reduced morning fatigue.

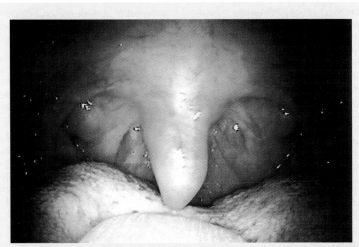

Case 6.1A Before

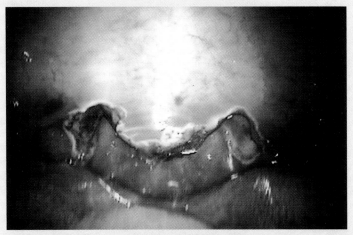

Case 6.1B One month after first LAUP.

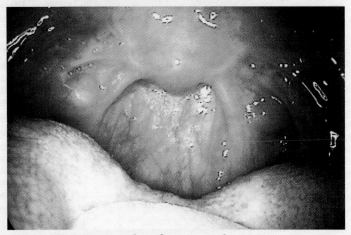

Case 6.1C Two months after second LAUP.

REFERENCES

1. Ikematsu T. Study of snoring, 4th report: therapy. *J Jpn Otol Rhionol Laryngol* 1964;64:434–5.
2. Lugaresi E, Cirignotta F, Coccagna G, et al. The relationship between snoring, smoking, body mass index, age, alcohol consumption, and respiratory symptoms. *Eur Respir J* 1989;2:599–603.
3. Fujita S. Method of Fujita. In: Fairbanks DNF, Fujita S, Ikematsu T, Simmons FB, eds. *Snoring and obstructive sleep apnea.* New York: Raven Press, 1987;134–53.
4. Koslenvuo M, Kaprio J, Partinen M, et al. Snoring as a risk factor for hypertension and angina pectoris. *Lancet* 1965;1:893–6.
5. Partinen M, Palomaki H. Snoring and cerebral infarction. *Lancet* 1985;2:1325–6.
6. Sher AE. Obstructive sleep apnea syndrome: a complex disorder of the upper airway. *Otolaryngol Clin North Am* 1990;23:593–608.
7. Guilleminault C, Telkian A, Dement W. Sleep apnea syndrome. *Am Rev Med* 1976;27:465–84.
8. Ferber R, Millman R, Coppola M, Fleetham J, et al. ASDA Standards of practice: portable recordings in the assessment of obstructive sleep apnea. *Sleep* 1994;17:378–92.
9. Rundell OH, Jones RK. Polysomnography methods and interpretations. *Otolaryngol Clin North Am* 1990;23:583–92.
10. Katsantonis GP, Schweitzer PK, Branham GH, et al. Management of obstructive sleep apnea: comparison of various treatment modalities. *Laryngoscope* 1988;98:304–9.
11. Maniglia AJ. Sleep apnea and snoring: an overview. *Ear Nose Throat J* 1993;72:16–9.
12. Kales A, Cadieux RJ, Bixler EO, et al. Severe OSA: onset, clinical course, and characteristics. *J Chronic Dis* 1985;38:419–25.
13. Lugaresi E, Cirignotta F, Cirignotta G, Piana D. Some epidemiologic data on snoring and cardiocirculatory disturbances. *Sleep* 1980;3:221–4.
14. Surrat PM, Dec P, Atkinson RL, Armstrong P, Wilholt SC. Fluoroscopic and computed tomographic features of pharyngeal airway in OSA. *Am Rev Respir Dis* 1983;127:487–92.
15. Haponik EF, Bohlman M, Smith PL, et al. CT scanning in OSA: correlation of structure with airway physiology during sleep and wakefulness. *Am Rev Respir Dis* 1982;125:107–13.
16. Ryan CF, Lowe AA, Li D, Fletham JA. Magnetic resonance imaging of the upper airway in OSA before and after chronic nasal continuous positive airway pressure treatment. *Am Rev Respir Dis* 1991;144:939–44.
17. Reiley R, Guilleminault C, Powell N, Simmons FB. Palatopharyngoplasty failure, cephalometric roentgenograms, and OSA. *Otolaryngol Head Neck Surg* 1985;93:240–3.
18. Woolfson BT, Wooten MR. Manometric and endoscopic localization of airway obstruction after uvulopalatopharyngoplasty. *Otolaryngol Head Neck Surg* 1994;11:38–43.
19. Rivlin J, Hoffstein V, Kalbfleisch J, et al. Upper airway morphology in patients with idiopathic OSA. *Am Rev Respir Dis* 1984;129:355–60.

20. Keidar A, Khosh M, Zammit G, Krespi Y. Self-reported symptoms and polysomnographic findings in laser-assisted uvulopalatoplasty patients. *Otolaryngol Head Neck Surg* (*submitted*).
21. Horner RL, Mohiaddin RH, Lowell DG, et al. Sites and sizes of fat deposits around the pharynx in obese patients with obstructive sleep apnea and weight-matched controls. *Eur Respir J* 1989;2:613–22.
22. Issa FG, Sullivan CE. Upper airway closing pressure in snorers. *J Appl Physiol* 1984;57:528–35.
23. Issa FG, Sullivan CE. Alcohol, snoring, and sleep apnea. *J Neurol Neurosurg Psychiatry* 1982;45:353–59.
24. Nino-Murcia G, McCann CC, Bliwise DL, et al. Compliance and side effects in sleep apnea patients treated with nasal continuous positive airway pressure. *West J Med* 1989;150:165–9.
25. Guilleminault C, Stoohs R, Clerk A, et al. A cause of excessive daytime sleepiness—the upper airway resistance syndrome. *Chest* 1993;104:781–7.
26. Sher AE. Obstructive sleep apnea syndrome: a complex disorder of the upper airway. *Otolaryngol Clin North Am* 1990;23:593–608.
27. Kamami YV. Laser CO_2 for snoring—preliminary results. *Acta Otolaryngol (Stockh)* 1990;44:451–6.
28. Krespi YP, Pearlman SJ, Keidar A, et al. Laser-assisted uvulopalatoplasty for snoring. *Insights Otolaryngol* 1994;9:1–8.
29. Krespi YP, Pearlman SJ, Keidar A. Laser-assisted uvulopalatoplasty for snoring. *J Otolaryngol* 1994;23:328–34.
30. Katsantonis GP, Friedman WH, Rosenblum BN, Walsh JK. The surgical treatment of snoring: a patient's perspective. *Laryngoscope* 1990;100:138–40.
31. Krespi YP, Keidar A, Khosh M, Pearlman SJ, Zammit G. The efficacy of laser uvulopalatoplasty in the management of obstructive sleep apnea syndrome and upper airway resistance syndrome. *Operative Techniques Otolaryngol Head Neck Surg* 1994;5:234–43.
32. Ellis PD, Williams JE, Shneerson JM. Surgical relief of snoring due to palatal flutter: a preliminary report. *Ann R Coll Surg Eng* 1993;75:286–90.
33. Carenfelt C. Laser uvulopalatoplasty in treatment of habitual snoring. *Ann Otol Rhinol Laryngol* 1991;100:451–4.
34. Sequert C, Carles P, Kamami PY, et al. Treatment of simple snoring. Surgical pharyngoplasty vs. laser CO_2 pharyngotomy. *Ann Otolaryngol Chir Cervicofac* 1992;109:317–22.
35. Fairbanks DN, Fujta S. Method of Coleman: laser-assisted uvulopalatoplasty. In: *Snoring and obstructive sleep apnea.* New York: Raven Press, 1994;136–45.

7
LASER TREATMENT
OF SCARS

Tina S. Alster, M.D.

7.1 INTRODUCTION

Hypertrophic scars and keloids affect an estimated 4.5–16% of the
population (1) and are notoriously difficult to treat. While more
deeply pigmented races appear to be especially susceptible, any
individual may develop a persistent hypertrophic scar or keloid following surgery or trauma. These types of scars are commonly
encountered in areas that typically demonstrate a slow wound-
healing response, such as the anterior chest, or in pressure or
movement-dependent areas, such as the scapula. By definition, a
hypertrophic scar is usually raised and erythematous but remains
within the confines of the original trauma. In contrast, a keloid is
more nodular and extends beyond the margins of the inciting
wound.

A variety of treatments for hypertrophic scars and keloids have
been advocated in the past, including intralesional steroids (2–5),
cryosurgery (5–7), radiotherapy (8–15), pressure therapy (16,17),
silicone gel sheeting (18–22), and excisional surgery (23–25). After
all these treatments, however, hypertrophic scars and keloids frequently recurred or even worsened.

Ablative laser surgical procedures utilizing carbon dioxide, argon,
and Nd:YAG lasers (26–33) were intermittently advocated in the past
as viable treatment options, but recurrences were common within 2

Cosmetic Laser Surgery, Edited by Alster, M.D. and Apfelberg, M.D.
ISBN 0471-12242-4   © 1996 Wiley-Liss, Inc.

years postoperatively. In contrast to the ablative properties of the aforementioned lasers, the 585 nm flashlamp-pumped pulsed dye laser (FPPDL) with a 450-μs pulse duration is specifically absorbed by hemoglobin-containing structures, effectively removing such microvascular lesions as telangiectasias and port-wine stains (38–41). In the past few years, it has been shown to improve the clinical appearance (color and height), cutaneous surface texture, pliability, and symptoms, such as pruritis and dysesthesia, of hypertrophic scars (34–37) without the recurrences noted with other laser systems.

7.2 FLASHLAMP-PUMPED PULSED DYE LASER (585-nm, 450-μs) PROTOCOL

While lighter skin tones (types I,II,III) absorb 585-nm wavelength light better due to less absorption by overlying epidermal melanin, any skin type could conceivably be treated with this laser system (Figure 7.1, Table 7.1). The entire scar is treated at each session with energy densities ranging between 6.5 and 7.25 J/cm^2 when using a 5-mm spot size and between 6.0 and 6.75 J/cm^2 with a 7-mm spot size. Immediately following laser irradiation, purpura lasting approximately 7–10 days appears within the scar. The skin is cleansed with mild soap and water and an antibiotic ointment is applied twice daily until the purpura resolves. The scar is evaluated at 6 or more weeks and, if erythema or hypertrophy is still evident, the scar is retreated using the same or slightly increased fluence.

While most hypertrophic scars show a mean improvement of 83% following two laser sessions (34), more fibrotic or keloid scars may require as many as six laser treatments to achieve the desired degree of lightening and flattening (T. Alster, *unpublished data*). Treatments are delivered at 6–8-week time intervals to allow for adequate dermal healing between laser exposures.

TABLE 7.1 Laser Protocol for Scars

- Skin types I–III best
- All body locations possible
- No anesthesia necessary
- Flashlamp-pumped pulsed dye laser (585-nm, 450-μs)
- Energy density of 6.0–7.5 J/cm^2
- Spot size of 5 or 7 mm
- Single, nonoverlapping laser pulses
- Treatment intervals of 6–8 weeks

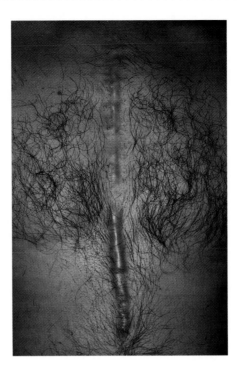

FIGURE 7.1 Keloid median sternotomy scar s/p two 585 nm flashlamp-pumped pulsed dye laser treatments to upper half only.

7.3 DISCUSSION

It has now been shown through controlled (37) (Table 7.2) and uncontrolled (case) studies (34–36) that the 585-nm flashlamp-pumped pulsed dye laser is effective in significantly improving the appearance of hypertrophic scars and keloids. Skin surface texture within laser-irradiated scars has been measured objectively using a computer-assisted digital imaging program (optical profilometry) and been shown to approximate the texture of normal skin within two laser treatments (34,35,37). Scar height and pliability are also significantly improved following laser treatment. Histologic examination of scar tissue shows the expected decrease in sclerotic collagen following laser irradiation.

TABLE 7.2 Flashlamp-Pumped Pulsed Dye Laser Treatment of Median Sternotomy Scars: A Controlled Study (37)

LASER-TREATED SCARS (2 TREATMENTS, 7 J/cm^2)	CONTROLS (NO TREATMENT)
• No symptoms (pruritis, burning)	• 75% symptomatic
• Reduced scar erythema	• No change in erythema
• Decreased scar height (1.37 mm)	• No reduced height (3.62 mm)
• Increased pliability	• No change in pliability
• Improved skin texture	• Same as baseline skin texture
• Looser, less coarse collagen	• Thick hyalinized collagen
• Increased number of mast cells	• Normal number of mast cells

The mechanism whereby hypertrophic and keloidal scars are altered by this vascular-specific laser system is unknown. Similar long-standing clinical results have not been obtained using lasers that merely vaporize or coagulate scar tissue, such as the continuous-wave carbon dioxide, Nd:YAG, and argon lasers (42–44). One may reasonably surmise that the specificity of the 585-nm pulsed dye laser for cutaneous microvessels is therefore important.

The 585-nm FPPDL laser affects skin by a process called "selective photothermolysis," a concept first described by Anderson and Parrish (45). Selective absorption of light by hemoglobin leads to local heating of cutaneous blood vessels, which is confined by use of a sufficiently short laser pulse duration. Irreversible, selective thermal injury of vessels leads to a process of thrombosis, vasculitis, and gradual local repair, including neovascularization (46). Little is known, however, about the influence of this process on ischemia, dermal metabolism, or control of the dermal extracellular matrix. Microvascular destruction by the laser presumably leads to a period of ischemia, which may affect collagen composition, metabolism, or release of collagenase. It is also possible that sufficient heat is conducted from blood vessels to the surrounding dermis to directly alter the collagen or other composition of the scar.

Perhaps the most likely explanation for this laser's effectiveness in the treatment of scars is related in some way to the increased number of dermal mast cells observed after treatment. Previous studies have demonstrated stimulation of normal and keloid fibroblast growth by histamine (47). While seemingly ambiguous, further investigations determining the role of mast cells in normal and scar tissue metabolism may provide a clue in the search for a reasonable mechanism of action for this particular laser treatment.

7.4 FURTHER TREATMENT TRENDS AND STUDIES

Previous reports on laser treatment of scars have been limited to those scars that already exist. Certainly, in those individuals who are prone to develop hypertrophic or keloid scars, it would seem reasonable to initiate laser treatment as early as possible after surgery or trauma in an attempt to prevent their eventual formation. While the optimal time for intervention remains unknown, most hypertrophic scars and keloids begin their development within the first 1–2 months following injury.

Most studies to date have limited their analyses to scars of several months' duration. Anecdotal reports (T. Alster, unpublished data) suggest that earlier intervention may produce better clinical improvement. The frequency with which laser treatments should be delivered to prevent scar formation or reverse existing scar tissue is another area requiring further study. Currently, the same FPPDL laser treatment parameters and intervals are used as in the treatment of vascular lesions. Treatment sessions at shorter intervals may yield improved results. In addition, the optimal energy densities to elicit the desired scar response need to be determined for different skin tones, body locations, and scar types. Lastly, the concomitant use of other treatments such as chemical peels, carbon dioxide laser resurfacing, corticosteroid injections, or topical formulations (i.e., silicone, retinoic acid) needs to be evaluated. It is suspected that combination therapies may provide quicker clinical improvement. These nebulous areas will undoubtedly be cleared as more investigations are completed on the laser treatment of scars.

CASE 7.1 ERYTHEMATOUS AND HYPERTROPHIC BREAST SCARS

A 30-year-old woman presented with erythematous and slightly hyper-trophic scars on her breasts following a breast augmentation procedure 1 year earlier (Case Figure 7.1A). She had noted apparent worsening of the scars within the first month after surgery and had failed to see any significant improvement in their appearance despite the use of silicone gel sheeting for 6 months.

Anesthesia: None

Procedure: Flashlamp-pumped pulsed dye laser (585 nm) laser treatment with a 7-mm spot size and 6.25 J/cm^2 fluence was delivered over the entire scar surface and repeated after 8 weeks.

Postoperative Care: Treated areas were cleansed with mild soap and water followed by antibiotic ointment twice daily until purpura resolved (7–10 days).

Postoperative Results: Scars showed significant improvement (Case Figure 7.1B) within 1 month following second laser treatment. No recurrence has been noted at 2-year follow-up examination.

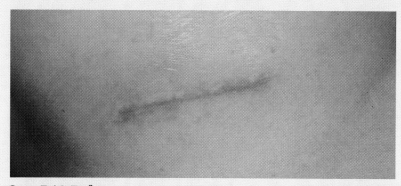

Case 7.1A Before

Case 7.1B After

CASE 7.2 ABDOMINAL SURGICAL SCAR

A 40-year-old woman desired treatment for a prominent scar on her abdomen after undergoing an exploratory laparotomy 2 years prior (Case Figure 7.2A). She complained of intermittent itching and burning within her scar. She had had intralesional corticosteroid injections which failed to alleviate her symptoms. Silicone gel sheeting had been applied for several months without noticeable improvement.

Anesthesia: None

Procedure: Three flashlamp-pumped pulsed dye laser treatments with a mean fluence of 6.75 J/cm^2 using nonoverlapping 5-mm spots over the entire scar at bimonthly intervals.

Postoperative Care: Twice daily cleansing with mild soap and water followed by antibiotic ointment and a nonstick bandage.

Postoperative Results: Patient showed marked improvement in the color, height, and texture of her scar (Case Figure 7.2B). Symptoms were alleviated immediately following the first laser treatment. No recurrence of scar or symptoms has been noted at 1-year follow-up examination.

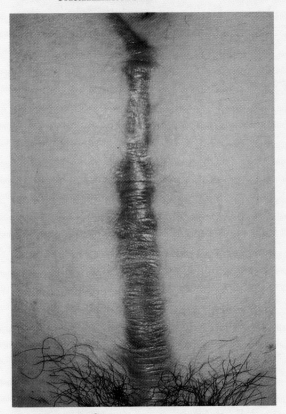

Case 7.2A Before

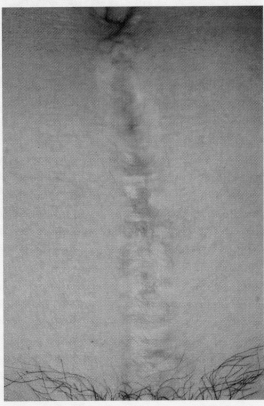

Case 7.2B After

CASE 7.3 FACIAL BURN SCARS

A 16-year-old boy developed hypertrophic scars on his cheeks, ears, and forehead after suffering burns from a gasoline explosion at the age of 8 (Case Figure 7.3A). He had had an operation to release scar contractures 1 year after his accident, but had not received any further treatments since that time.

Anesthesia: None

Procedure: Three flashlamp-pumped pulsed dye laser treatments delivered at 8-week intervals using fluences ranging from 6.0 to 6.5 J/cm^2 with a 5–7-mm spot size.

Postoperative Care: Daily cleansing with soap and water and application of antibiotic ointment.

Postoperative Results: Marked reduction in scar erythema and scar height (Case Figure 7.3B). Patient was able to shave without nicking and was no longer self-conscious. No recurrence noted at 18-month follow-up.

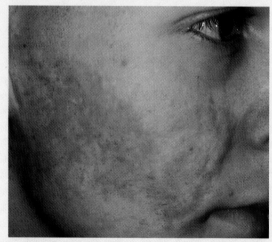

Case 7.3A Before

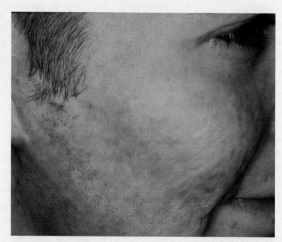

Case 7.3B After

CASE 7.4 ATROPHIC ACNE SCARS

A 35-year-old woman with a long-standing history of acne presented with subsequent scar development over her cheeks (Case Figure 7.4A). No prior dermabrasion or other scar treatment had been performed.

Anesthesia: None

Procedure: One flashlamp-pumped pulsed dye laser treatment at 6.25 J/cm^2 using a 7-mm spot size on all cheek scars.

Postoperative Care: Twice daily antibiotic ointment applied after gentle cleansing with soap and water.

Postoperative Results: Erythematous component of atrophic scars completely resolved and skin surface texture improved by 50% (Case Figure 7.4B). Patient may consider future skin resurfacing procedure using a high-energy pulsed carbon dioxide laser for further improvement of her remaining atrophic scars.

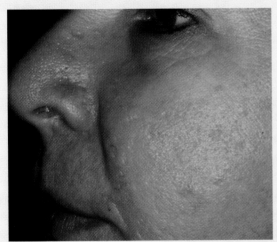

Case 7.4A Before

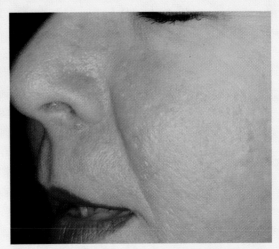

Case 7.4B After

REFERENCES

1. Cosman B, Crikelair GF, Ju DM, et al. The surgical treatment of keloids. *Plast Reconstr Surg* 1961;27:335–41.
2. Ketchum LD, Smith J, Robinson DW, Masters FW. Treatment of hypertrophic scar, keloids, and scar contracture by triamcinolone acetonide. *Plast Reconstr Surg* 1966;38:209–15.
3. Maguire HC Jr. Treatment of keloids with triamcinolone acetonide injected intralesionally. *JAMA* 1965;192:325–30.
4. Golladay ES. Treatment of keloids by single intraoperative perilesional injection of repository steroid. *South Med J* 1988;81:736–8.
5. Layton AM, Yip J, Cunliffe WJ. A comparison of intralesional triamcinolone and cryosurgery in the treatment of acne keloids. *Br J Dermatol* 1994;130:498–501.
6. Zouboulis CC, Blume U, Buttner P, Orfanos CE. Outcomes of cryosurgery in keloids and hypertrophic scars. A prospective consecutive trial of case series. *Arch Dermatol* 1993;129:1146–51.
7. Shepherd JP, Dawber RP. The response of keloid scars to cryosurgery. *Plast Reconstr Surg* 1982;70:677–82.
8. Klumpar DI, Murray JC, Anscher M. Keloids treated with excision followed by radiation therapy. *J Am Acad Dermatol* 1994;31:225–31.
9. Ship AG, Weiss PR, Mincer FR, Wolkstein W. Sternal keloids: successful treatment employing surgery and adjunctive radiation. *Ann Plast Surg* 1993;31:481–7.
10. Lo TC, Seckel BR, Salzman FA, Wright KA. Single–dose electron beam irradiation in the treatment and prevention of keloids and hypertrophic scars. *Radiother Oncol* 1990;19:267–72.
11. Sallstrom KO, Larson O, Heden P, et al. Treatment of keloids with surgical excision and postoperative x-ray radiation. *Scand J Plast Surg Hand Surg* 1989;23:211–5.
12. Borok TL, Bray M, Sinclair I, et al. Role of ionizing irradiation for 393 keloids. *J Radiat Oncol Biol Phys* 1988;15:865–70.
13. Ollstein RN, Siegel HW, Gillooley JF, Barsa JM. Treatment of keloids by combined surgical excision and immediate postoperative x-ray therapy. *Ann Plast Surg* 1981;7:281–5.
14. Lukacs S, Braun-Falco O, Goldschmidt H. Radiotherapy of benign dermatoses: indications, practice, and results. *J Dermatol Surg Oncol* 1978;4:620–5.
15. Craig RD, Pearson D. Early postoperative irradiation in the treatment of keloid scars. *Br J Plast Surg* 1965;18:369–76.
16. Carr-Collins JA. Pressure techniques for the prevention of hypertrophic scar. *Clin Plast Surg* 1992;19:733–43.
17. Ward RS. Pressure therapy for the control of hypertrophic scar formation after burn injury. A history and review. *J Burn Care Rehabil* 1991;12:257–62.
18. Gold MH. Topical silicone gel sheeting in the treatment of hypertrophic scars and keloids. A dermatologic experience. *J Dermatol Surg Oncol* 1993;19:912–6.
19. Sproat JE, Dalcin A, Weitauer N, Roberts RS. Hypertrophic sternal scars: silicone gel sheet versus kenalog injection treatment. *Plast Reconstr Surg* 1992;90:988–92.

20. Ahn ST, Monafo WW, Mustoe TA. Topical silicone gel for the prevention and treatment of hypertrophic scar. *Arch Surg* 1991;126:499–504.

21. Sawada Y, Sone K. Treatment of scars and keloids with a cream containing silicone oil. *Br J Plast Surg* 1990;43:683–8.

22. Mercer NS. Silicone gel in the treatment of keloid scars. *Br J Plast Surg* 1989;42:83–7.

23. Brown LA, Pierce HE. Keloids: scar revision. *J Dermatol Surg Oncol* 1986;12:51–6.

24. Pollack SV, Goslen JB. The surgical treatment of keloids. *J Dermatol Surg Oncol* 1982;8:1045–9.

25. Apfelberg DB, Maser MR, Lash H. The use of epidermis over a keloid as an autograft after resection of the keloid. *J Dermatol Surg Oncol* 1976;2:409–15.

26. Lim TC, Tan WT. Carbon dioxide laser for keloids. *Plast Reconstr Surg* 1991;88:1111.

27. Sherman R, Rosenfeld H. Experience with the Nd:YAG laser in the treatment of keloid scars. *Ann Plast Surg* 1988;21:231–5.

28. Apfelberg DB, Smith T, Lash H, et al. Preliminary report on the use of the neodymium-YAG laser in plastic surgery. *Lasers Surg Med* 1987;7:189–98.

29. Hulsbergen-Henning JP, Roskam Y, van Gemert MJ. Treatment of keloids and hypertrophic scars with an argon laser. *Lasers Surg Med* 1986;6:72–5.

30. Kantor GR, Wheeland RG, Bailin PL, et al. Treatment of earlobe keloids with carbon dioxide laser excision: a report of 16 cases. *J Dermatol Surg Oncol* 1985;11:1063–7.

31. Abergel RP, Dwyer RM, Meeker CA, et al. Laser treatment of keloids: a clinical trial and an in vitro study with Nd:YAG laser. *Lasers Surg Med* 1984;4:291–5.

32. Apfelberg DB, Maser MR, Lash H, et al. Preliminary results of argon and carbon dioxide laser treatment of keloid scars. *Lasers Surg Med* 1984;4:283–90.

33. Henderson DL, Cromwell TA, Mes LG. Argon and carbon dioxide laser treatment of hypertrophic and keloid scars. *Lasers Surg Med* 1984;3:271–7.

34. Alster TS. Improvement of erythematous and hypertrophic scars by the 585 nm flashlamp-pumped pulsed dye laser. *Ann Plast Surg* 1994;32:186–90.

35. Alster TS, Kurban AK, Grove GL, et al. Alteration of argon laser-induced scars by the pulsed dye laser. *Lasers Surg Med* 1993;13:368–73.

36. Dierickx C, Goldman MP, Fitzpatrick RE. Laser treatment of erythematous/hypertrophic and pigmented scars in 26 patients. *Plast Reconstr Surg* 1995;95:84–90.

37. Alster TS, Williams CM. Improvement of hypertrophic and keloidal median sternotomy scars by the 585 nm flashlamp-pumped pulsed dye laser: a controlled study. *Lancet* 1995;345:1198–200.

38. Alster TS, Wilson F. Treatment of portwine stains with the 585 nm flashlamp-pumped pulsed dye laser: extended clinical experience. *Ann Plast Surg* 1994;32:478–84.

39. Alster TS, Tan OT. Laser treatment of benign cutaneous vascular lesions. *Am Fam Physician* 1991;44:547–54.

40. Tan OT, Sherwood K, Gilchrest BA. Treatment of children with port-wine stains using the flashlamp-pulsed tunable dye laser. *N Engl J Med* 1989;320:416–21.

41. Anderson RR, Parrish JA. Microvasculature can be selectively damaged using dye lasers: a basic theory and experimental evidence in human skin. *Lasers Surg Med* 1981;1:263–76.

42. Norris JE. The effect of carbon dioxide laser surgery on the recurrence of keloids. *Plast Reconstr Surg* 1991;87:44–9.

43. Stern JC, Lucente FE. Carbon dioxide laser excision of earlobe keloids. A prospective study and critical analysis of existing data. *Arch Otolaryngol Head Neck Surg* 1989;115:1107–11.

44. Apfelberg DB, Maser MR, White DN, Lash H. Failure of carbon dioxide laser excision of keloids. *Lasers Surg Med* 1989;9:382–8.

45. Anderson RR, Parrish JA. Selective photothermolysis: precise microsurgery by selective absorption of pulsed radiation. *Science* 1983;220:524–7.

46. Nakagawa H, Tan OT, Parrish JA. Ultrastructural changes in human skin after exposure to pulsed laser. *J Invest Dermatol* 1985;84:396–400.

47. Topol BM, Lewis VL Jr, Benveniste K. The use of antihistamine to retard the growth of fibroblasts derived from human skin, scar, and keloid. *Plast Reconstr Surg* 1981;68:231–2.

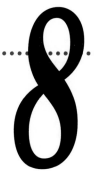

LASER TREATMENT
OF TELANGIECTASIAS

Heidi A. Waldorf, M.D.

Gary P. Lask, M.D.

Roy G. Geronemus, M.D.

8.1 INTRODUCTION

A telangiectasia is a permanently dilated cutaneous blood vessel visible to the naked eye (1). Telangiectasias are common cutaneous findings estimated to occur in up to 48% of healthy children and 15% of normal adults (2,3). Telangiectasias of the lower extremities occur in 29–41% of women and 6–15% of men (4). Although these figures suggest that childhood telangiectasias regress, spontaneous involution usually does not occur (5). The incidence increases with the impact of intrinsic and extrinsic factors on the skin (Table 8.1).

Telangiectasias occur as single or multiple vessels. By definition, individual vessel diameter does not exceed 0.1–1 millimeter (mm) (6). The clinical appearance of the vessel can be a clue to its origin. Wiry, red telangiectasias generally extend from arterioles or from the arterial side of a capillary loop. Cordlike, blue vessels arise from venules or from the venous side of a capillary loop. Red telangiectasias arising in the capillary loop may also become more blue with time as hydrostatic pressure and venous backflow increase (6).

Telangiectasias have also been classified by clinical pattern (7). Sinus or simple telangiectasias are linear red or blue vessels that arise from capillaries, most commonly on the midface and lower extremities. Arborizing telangiectasias appear to extend in the direc-

---

Cosmetic Laser Surgery, Edited by Alster, M.D. and Apfelberg, M.D.
ISBN 0471-12242-4 © 1996 Wiley-Liss, Inc.

TABLE 8.1   Etiologic Factors of Telangiectasias

INTRINSIC	EXTRINSIC
Genetic or congenital	Drug-induced
Vascular nevi	Estrogen
Genetic syndromes	Corticosteroids
Bloom's syndrome	
Rothmund–Thomson syndrome	Actinic dermatitis
Primary cutaneous disorders	Radiation dermatitis
Rosacea	
Poikiloderma of Civatte	Postsurgical
	Rhinoplasty
	Wound closure under tension
Systemic disease	
Collagen vascular disease	
Cushing's disease	
Metastatic carcinoma	Postsclerotherapy
Other	Traumatic
Pregnancy	
Venous incompetence	

tion of venous flow. Histologic examination of blue arborizing vessels on the legs has revealed that they represent dilated venules or ectatic veins, possibly with direct connections to underlying larger veins (2,8,9). Spider or star telangiectasias, in the past called "spider nevi," are composed of red radiating arms extending outward from a central pulsating arteriole (10). Centrally applied pressure produces centrifugal blanching. These vessels are commonly seen as an isolated acquired lesion in children, most often over the dorsum of the hands, forearms, and face, and in adults, on the face, neck, and thorax (2,11). Punctiform or papular telangiectasias may be seen as a component of genetic syndromes, such as generalized essential telangiectasia (12), and collagen vascular diseases, such as progressive systemic sclerosis (13).

The development of these vessels is a reflection of capillary or venular neogenesis induced by vasoactive factors (6). The release or activation of these substances can be triggered by exogenous or endogenous chemicals including alcohol, estrogens, and corticosteroids (14–16). Direct physical factors also play an important role. Chronic actinic exposure results in direct damage to the microcirculation as well as massive loss of the supporting connective tissue matrix (17). In rosacea, frequent vasodilation of the superficial papillary plexus may decrease vascular tone and result in additional telangiectasias (18,19). Similarly, increased hydrostatic pressure in the venous system of the lower extremities induces persistent venous dilation, increased venular distensibility, and permanent telangiectasias (20). Postoperative and traumatic telangiectasias are an exaggeration of the normal revascularization that occurs during healing (21). In wounds under tension, anoxia-induced angiogenesis and skin atrophy increase the development of telangiectasias (22,23).

Although patients usually seek medical treatment for telangiectasias due to their unsightly appearance, telangiectasias are not merely a cosmetic problem. When papular, an individual telangiectasia may bleed with minor trauma (24). Dense clusters of telangiectasias, such as those seen in acne rosacea, contribute to flushing reactions that are socially stigmatizing and that may further exacerbate vascular dilation and inflammation (18,19,25). Telangiectasias of the legs may lead to burning, painful, or pruritic sensations with changes of temperature or with menses (26). As mentioned previously, the presence of numerous telangiectasias may be a marker of acquired and congenital dermatologic and internal disease.

Thus, telangiectasias can result in both cosmetic and functional problems for patients. Treatment of fine facial telangiectasias had been limited to electrodesiccation using very low amperage current (27,28). The vessel must be penetrated every 2–3 mm and, as a result of heat generation, superficial necrosis always occurs to some degree (24). Although excellent results may be achieved in experienced hands, electrosurgery is not consistently effective and has a relatively high risk of scarring. Sclerotherapy, which involves injection of a substance into the dilated vessel to induce fibrosis, is currently the standard treatment for telangiectasias of the lower extremities (29). Side effects may include the development of telangiectatic matting, hyperpigmentation, and ulceration (30,31). Although sclerotherapy has also been used for telangiectatic vessels on the face, the risk of complications is increased (24). In recent years, the treatment of telangiectasias has benefitted from advancing laser technology. In this chapter, the background biophysics and practical application of laser therapy of cutaneous telangiectasias are discussed.

8.2 CONTINUOUS-WAVE LASERS

A variety of continuous-wave (CW) and quasipulsed lasers are presently being used to treat facial telangiectasias. The wavelengths vary from 488 to 578 nm. The target chromophore is oxyhemoglobin. The longer wavelength lasers (yellow light at 577–585 nm) have the advantage of deeper penetration as well as greater selectivity of oxyhemoglobin versus melanin.

Facial telangiectasias are one of the most common conditions treated by cutaneous lasers. Their sizes range from 0.1 to 3 mm, with the vast majority measuring between 100 and 200 μm in diameter. The CW vascular laser is an excellent modality for the treatment of facial telangiectasias, especially larger caliber vessels, as compared to pulsed vascular lasers. Pulsed dye lasers, which emit yellow light, have pulse durations of approximately 450 microseconds (μs). This pulse width is matched to the thermal relaxation time of a median vessel size of 50–100 μm (the average vessel width seen in a port-wine stain) and is thus ideal in treating vessels contained within macular port-wine stains or small facial telangiectasias, but not larger caliber vessels.

8.2.1 Argon Laser

The argon laser was the first CW laser used to treat telangiectasias (32). It emits light at six different wavelengths from 458 to 514 nm with 80% of its emission at 488 nm and 514.5 nm (33,34). The argon laser has the ability to be pulsed with a shuttering mechanism.

For several years, the argon laser was the customary laser for the treatment of vascular lesions. Presently, it is used primarily to treat vascular lesions containing large caliber vessels or larger caliber telangiectasias. As with other CW lasers, when treating vascular lesions, the laser light penetrates through the epidermis and is absorbed by hemoglobin. The light is then converted to heat, resulting in thermal coagulation of the blood vessels. Histopathology has confirmed some degree of vessel destruction occurring as deep as 1 mm in the dermis (35,36). Facial telangiectasias are thus quite amenable to argon laser treatment. In one study, 42 out of 50 patients treated experienced complete blanching without scar or recurrence after one laser application (37).

The treatment of facial telangiectasias by CW lasers is performed without the use of local anesthesia. The argon laser is delivered through a fiber optic cable using a pulse duration of 50 ms to 0.3 second and an energy of 0.8–2.9 watts, with spot sizes of 0.1 and 1 mm (38).

Following argon laser treatment, minimal crusting usually occurs, which resolves within 5–10 days. Scarring, although rare in the treatment of facial telangiectasias, certainly can occur, as well as pigment alteration. Despite the affinity for laser light absorption by oxyhemoglobin, nonselective thermal damage can take place with the use of the argon laser.

One of the limiting factors of the argon laser is its depth of penetration. Since thermal injury is limited to the upper 1 mm of the dermis, the laser is most effective for the treatment of superficial papillary dermal lesions. In treating tanned or darkly pigmented skin, the absorption of melanin in the epidermis by the argon laser decreases laser light penetration, which subsequently prevents significant absorption by hemoglobin and leads to increased risk of permanent pigmentary alteration.

8.2.2 Argon-Pumped Tunable Dye Laser

The argon-pumped tunable dye laser (APTDL) is a CW laser with the capability of being pulsed at pulse widths as short as 30 ms using a shuttering mechanism (39). The emitting laser uses various organic dyes, each of which can cover an expected range of about 50–1200 nm. This light is filtered by way of a prism or tuning wedge, which subsequently allows for a band of monochromatic light at the selected wavelength (40). This particular laser source is able to emit coherent light at virtually any wavelength, from blue to near-infrared.

The APTDL is presently being used at 577 nm and at variable spot sizes in the treatment of telangiectasias. The beam is transmitted through a fiber optic cable with a small spot size and relatively low power output, yielding high-energy densities. Treating facial telangiectasias with the tracing technique requires a spot size as small as 100 μm and a loop magnification of 3× to 8×. Using a 100-μm spot size, the APTDL is set at pulses of 0.05–0.1 second for continuous hand tracing. Power settings are usually set at 0.1–0.4 watt and the wavelength is adjusted to 577–585 nm (41). Because energy is focused into a very small spot size, the power settings at 0.1 and 0.2 watt have power densities of 1000–2000 watts/cm^2. A threshold blanching is observed with treatment. Postoperatively, erythema and edema are observed (39).

A robotized scanner (hexascan) can be used for treating small diffuse telangiectasias. When comparing the hexascan using yellow (585 nm) and green (532 nm) wavelengths, comparable clinical results have been obtained at similar fluences (42,43). A pulse width of 30–100 ms is used with fluences of 18–20 joules/cm^2 (J/cm^2) for smaller diameter vessels and 22–30 J/cm^2 for larger dimensional vessels (44,45). In general, ectatic vessels of the caliber ranging from 30 to 300 μm should be amenable to APTDL therapy.

8.2.3 KTP Laser

The KTP laser is a CW laser that can be pulsed using a shuttering mechanism. The KTP laser uses a Nd:YAG crystal (1064 nm), which then is frequency-doubled using a potassium titanyl phosphate crystal to half the wavelength, thereby creating a 532-nm beam with characteristics similar to the argon laser.

The KTP laser can be very effective for the treatment of facial telangiectasias. This laser can also be used by way of a hexascanner delivery device to distribute a uniform energy dose in a hexagonal pattern. The hexascanner is best used for the treatment of large confluent telangiectatic areas. The energies used for treatment range from 10 to 18 joules/cm^2 (46). The shortest pulse possible is used in order to diminish the pain.

Treatment of linear telangiectasias can be performed using a 100-, 150-, or 250-μm handpiece. The 250-μm handpiece is commonly used for telangiectasias at 0.5–0.7 watt and a repeat pulse of 0.1 second on and 0.1 second off.

8.2.4 Copper Vapor Laser

The copper vapor laser emits yellow light at 578 nm. This laser, which was initially used for fingerprint identification and for military applications (47), can be used to treat facial telangiectasias. One study comparing the efficacy of the copper vapor laser with the argon-pumped tunable dye laser showed comparable clinical results (48). Although the copper vapor laser can also be configured to produce a wavelength at 511 nm, vascular lesions are best treated at 578 nm. Because the copper vapor laser emits light at 30–50 nanosecond (ns) pulses between 6000 and 15,000 times per second, it effectively acts likes a continuous-wave laser (40).

A 150-μm handpiece is used when treating facial telangiectasias utilizing an average power of 450–500 milliwatts (mW). The light is chopped by an electronic shutter at 0.2-second exposure intervals. Visual magnification of 3.5× to 6× is recommended (49,50).

8.2.5 Krypton Laser

The krypton laser is a CW laser that can emit yellow (568–577 nm) and green (520–530 nm) light through a shuttering mechanism. Vascular lesions are treated with the yellow light and the beam is delivered through a fiber optic cable. The treatment of facial telangiectasias is usually performed utilizing a 100-μm collimated or a 1-mm handpiece. The parameters are set at 0.4–0.6 watt with a 0.2-second pulsed or continuous wave when using a 100-μm handpiece and 0.7–0.9 watt with a 0.2-second pulsed or continuous wave when using a 1-mm handpiece. The treatment endpoints and possible complications are the same as for other CW vascular lasers.

8.2.6 Copper Bromide Laser

The copper bromide laser has a wavelength of 578-nm as well as a wavelength of 511 nm. The 578-nm wavelength is used to treat vascular lesions. The machine is a quasipulsed laser using pulses as short as 7 ms. The laser is emitted at 16 kilohertz (kHz). The light is delivered through a fiber optic cable with a spot size of 0.7 mm when focused 1 mm from the skin surface. It is an excellent machine for facial telangiectasias composed of larger caliber vessels.

8.3 PULSED LASERS

8.3.1 Flashlamp-Pumped Pulsed Dye Laser

The flashlamp-pumped pulsed dye laser (PDL) was developed specifically for the treatment of cutaneous vascular lesions. The wavelength of the PDL was initially set at 577 nm, corresponding to an absorption peak of oxyhemoglobin. The wavelength has since been increased to 585 nm, which provides for a greater depth of dermal penetration with similar vascular selectivity (51). Based on the theory of selective photothermolysis, the PDL pulse duration of 450 μs is shorter than the 1–5 ms thermal relaxation time of superficial cutaneous blood vessels (52,53). Each laser pulse ends before heat can diffuse to adjacent structures, thus confining damage to the target vessels.

Originally studied on port-wine stain lesions, histologic evaluation confirmed the theoretical benefits of the PDL over CW lasers. Laser-treated papillary and upper reticular dermal vessels reveal agglutination of erythrocytes and vessel wall degeneration to a depth of 1.2 mm (51,53). Fine granulation tissue replaces the damaged vessels after 1 week. Histology at 1 month shows a normal-appearing dermis and epidermis with fine capillaries and normal adnexal structures without fibrosis. Clinically, these changes correlate with a 7–14 day period of post-treatment purpura with partial

or complete vessel clearance without scarring at 1 month. These
findings are the basis for the minimum 4-week interval between
PDL treatment sessions (Figures 8.1 and 8.2).

In addition to requiring the appropriate wavelength and pulse
duration for the target lesion, these laser–tissue interactions are

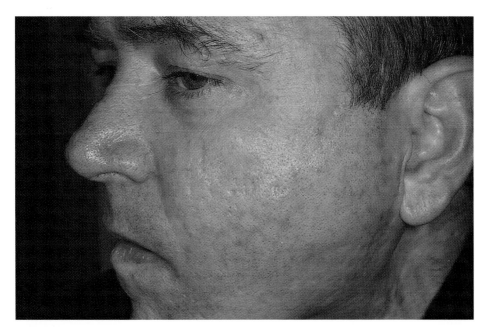

FIGURE 8.1 Lattice-like effect of treated and untreated skin 1 month following pulsed dye laser treatment of diffuse telangiectasias (6 J/cm^2, 7-mm
spot size).

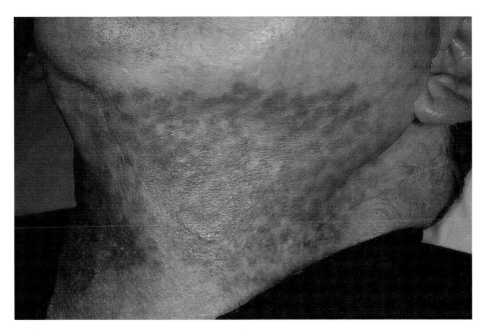

FIGURE 8.2 Immediate purpura following pulsed dye laser treatment of
diffuse telangiectasia of the neck (5.25 J/cm^2, 7-mm spot size).

dependent on other parameters. Absorption of laser light of a given wavelength is varied by changing the spot size of the beam. The PDL is currently available with handpieces that deliver 2-, 3-, 5-, and 7-mm diameter beams. Fluence, the total energy per unit area, ranges therapeutically from 5 to 9 J/cm^2 (34). Since reducing spot size decreases the effective energy delivered, a higher fluence is required to produce the same result when a smaller beam is used. In addition, because melanin interferes with absorption of the PDL pulses, energy delivery will be greater through less pigmented skin (38). The clinical response to a test pulse can be used as a gauge. Suitable laser settings should produce purpura without excessive edema, crusting, blistering, or other epidermal change.

The PDL is useful for a variety of telangiectatic lesions. The location and morphology of the lesion being treated determine the initial parameters of the PDL. Over 70% of spider telangiectasias of the face in children and 93% in adults clear after one PDL treatment using fluences of 6.0–7.5 J/cm^2 with a 5-mm spot size (5,54). Higher fluences should be reserved for older children, adults, or subsequent treatment of resistent vessels. In lesions smaller than the spot size used, one pulse to the central punctum of the spider telangiectasia is all that is necessary. The lesion should become purpuric immediately and should no longer blanch with pressure. Radiating vessels not covered by the initial pulse are treated with subsequent pulses with 0–10% overlap. Smaller spot sizes have the advantage of reduced purpura, but, to be effective, higher fluences of 8.5–10 J/cm^2 must be used (24,38).

Other forms of facial telangiectasias respond well to the PDL but are more likely to require more than one treatment session. Linear telangiectasias, such as those frequently found around the nasal ala, are less likely to show skin texture changes with the PDL than with the other lasers. In one series, 97.5% of these patients had more than 50% vessel clearance after one or two treatments (55). This study showed the most favorable responses with fluences above 7 J/cm^2. Larger blue vessels respond less well than smaller red vessels, due to a longer thermal relaxation time and a higher ratio of deoxygenated to oxygenated hemoglobin in the former (56). A new handpiece currently under study produces an elliptical-shaped beam designed to optimize the treatment of linear vessels (Candela Laser Corp., Wayland, MA).

Patients with diffuse facial telangiectasias seen as a component of rosacea, actinic damage, and chronic corticosteroid use can have excellent cosmetic results with the PDL. Indeed, there is some evidence to suggest that even the inflammatory (pustular and papular) component of rosacea is decreased following PDL treatment of associated telangiectasias (57). In addition, the incidence of flushing induced by vasodilation of telangiectatic vessels is reduced. The widespread telangiectatic component of certain genetic syndromes, such as Rothmund–Thomson (58) and Goltz's (59) syndromes, has been treated with similar success. Clearance of large areas of interlacing vessels is best achieved using larger spot sizes (5 or 7 mm) with fluences of $6.0-7.5$ J/cm^2 (57). Since the majority of these patients are fair-skinned, lower fluences may be adequate. Although some authors advocate overlapping spots $10-33\%$, the risk of epidermal damage, which can lead to textural changes or scar formation, is reduced significantly when pulses are *not* overlapped. Patients must be advised prior to the procedure that additional sessions will be necessary to clear the lattice of vessels remaining between adjacent pulses.

Treatment of nonfacial telangiectasias requires special attention to the lesion site. Poikiloderma of Civatte is a photodistributed reticulated telangiectatic network with associated hyperpigmentation and dermal atrophy involving primarily the neck and upper chest (60). The PDL has been used effectively to clear the erythema in these areas at fluences of $6.5-7.0$ J/cm^2 after an average of four treatment sessions (61). Because the neck and chest are particularly susceptible to adverse side effects, it is important to evaluate a test treatment at a low energy fluence prior to treating a large area. Generalized essential telangiectasia, a progressive disorder characterized by netlike, noninflamed dilated vessels, particularly on the lower extremities, has been treated similarly (38,62).

As described, the treatment of telangiectasias with the PDL is safe and effective with minimal incidence of adverse sequelae. Each laser pulse causes a rubberband-like, snapping sensation that is generally quite tolerable without anesthesia. The major disadvantage of the PDL technique is the transient purpura, which may be difficult to camouflage in the initial days following treatment. Thus patients must be forewarned so that they can schedule their treatments accordingly. The most common epidermal changes following PDL treatment of telangiectasias are scaling and crusting, which occurs in 12% and 4% of cases, respectively (38). Blistering and scarring are seen in less than 1% of cases and are usually associated with using energy densities that are too high for a given area or lesion. Pigmentary changes are also infrequent and generally resolve spontaneously within several months. These changes are more common when treating darker skin tones or suntanned skin. Utilizing the lowest effective fluences and minimizing pulse overlapping reduce the risk of side effects.

Laser treatment of leg telangiectasias has posed a more difficult challenge. Laser treatment has theoretical advantages over standard sclerotherapy. Telangiectatic matting and hyperpigmentation are estimated to occur in up to 30% of sclerotherapy patients (4). However, early attempts to treat lower extremity telangiectasias with the PDL were disappointing, with less improvement and more and longer-lasting hypo- and hyperpigmentation than that observed after laser treatment of other sites (63). More recent attempts to define the usefulness of the PDL for leg telangiectasias have had more success (4,38). It appears that the PDL may play a therapeutic role in the treatment of red telangiectasias less than 0.2 mm in diameter, including postsclerotherapy telangiectatic matting. Therapy is most effective if associated varicose and reticular feeding vessels are treated first. Because lower extremity telangiectasias are generally venules of larger caliber and with thicker walls than telangiectasias elsewhere, it has been hypothesized that a longer pulse duration of 1–10 ms may be required to damage the vessel wall. Such "long-pulse" PDLs are currently undergoing clinical trials (38) (Candela Laser Corp., Wayland, MA). Another pulsed light source that produces a noncoherent beam that includes a wide spectrum of wavelengths from 500 to 1100 nm (Photoderm VL, Energy Systems Corp., Needham, MA) is also under investigation for the treatment of leg vessels. The inclusion of longer wavelengths theoretically should provide deeper penetration of target vessels and improve absorption by the deoxyhemoglobin that predominates in venules (38,64).

8.4 SUMMARY

Multiple continuous-wave (CW) lasers have been used in the treatment of facial telangiectasias with excellent results and minimal complications. When comparison studies have been performed, primarily between continuous-wave (CW) and pulsed dye laser (PDL) treatment of facial telangiectasias, the majority of results have been equivocal. The advantage of the PDL, in general, is that the treatment times are shorter due to the larger spot size utilized. However, if smaller spot sizes are used to decrease the incidence of purpura, the treatment times become comparable. Certainly, the limiting factor of the PDL is the postoperative purpura that lasts, on average, 7-10 days. Patients thus tend to better tolerate the erythema and mild edema with subsequent minimal scabbing resulting from CW laser therapy. In general, discomfort usually is less with the CW lasers, probably as a result of the smaller spot sizes used. When a smaller spot size is used in conjunction with PDL treatment, similar pain is produced.

In one comparison study, the PDL was found to be more efficacious than the argon-pumped tunable dye laser (APTDL) in the overall treatment of facial telangiectasias (64). These results have not been corroborated by other comparative studies, suggesting that the findings may, in fact, be due to the operator-dependent techniques that are so important with CW laser use. In the study, there was no scarring, atrophy, or persistent textural changes noted following either treatment; however, transient postinflammatory hyperpigmentation was more common following PDL treatment. The reason for the differences seen may be attributed to the tendency of the APTDL to obscure adjacent telangiectasias during treatment, thereby causing them to be missed. In addition, the larger spot size of the PDL may also have contributed to the superior results observed due to a more thorough destruction of vessels.

In general, both CW and pulsed vascular lasers yield excellent results for facial telangiectasias with minimal complications. Pulsed dye lasers are best used for small caliber vessels and continuous-wave lasers for large caliber vessels. One exception may be in the treatment of extensive small facial telangiectasias, such as those seen in rosacea or actinically damaged skin. Use of the PDL requires a series of treatment sessions before complete clearing is achieved due to the lattice-pattern produced as a result of partial (erythematous) and full (skin-toned) vessel ablation. As such, some patients may prefer CW laser treatment to diminish only the most prominent vasculature while leaving background erythema. For delicate tissue areas (notably the anterior chest), the PDL yields excellent cosmetic results while minimizing side effects. The most efficacious laser treatment for leg telangiectasias is yet to be determined; however, longer pulse durations and wavelengths may allow for deeper penetration of laser light with superior clinical results.

CASE 8.1 TELANGIECTASIAS OF THE CHEEKS

A 35-year-old woman complained of facial redness that had been worsening over the previous 2 years (Case Figure 8.1A). No prior treatment had been received.

Diagnosis: Essential telangiectasias of the cheeks.

Procedure: A 585-nm flashlamp-pumped pulsed dye laser (PDL) at 7.0 J/cm^2 and 5-mm spot size was used for small caliber telangiectasias and diffuse background erythema.

Continuous-wave tunable dye laser (585 nm) with 0.1-mm spot and 0.8-watt power was used on the large caliber vessels. There were a total of two treatment sessions.

Postoperative Care: The patient applied bacitracin ointment twice daily during the 7–10 day healing phase.

Postoperative Results: Total resolution of her lesions was noted within 2 weeks following the second laser treatment (Case Figure 8.1B).

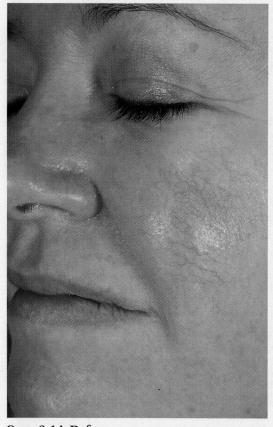 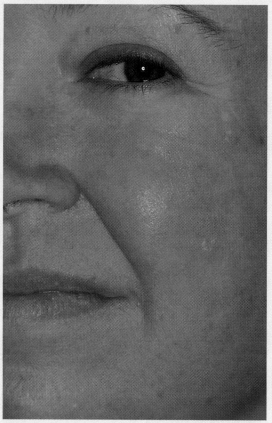

Case 8.1A Before   Case 8.1B After

CASE 8.2 ROSACEA OF CHEEKS AND NOSE

A 58-year-old woman complained of facial flushing for several years which was aggravated by extreme temperature changes, alcohol, caffeine, and spicy foods (Case Figure 8.2A). The patient had been placed on tetracycline and Metrogel without apparent benefit.

Diagnosis: Rosacea involving the cheeks and nose.
Anesthesia: None.
Procedure: A 585-nm flashlamp-pumped pulsed dye laser (PDL) with 7-mm spot size and 6.25 J/cm^2 was employed.
Postoperative Results: Patient no longer complained of flushing within 3 weeks following one laser treatment (Case Figure 8.2B).

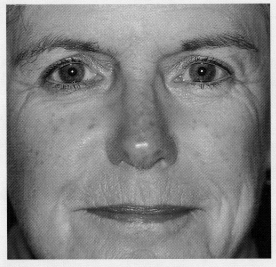

Case 8.2A Before

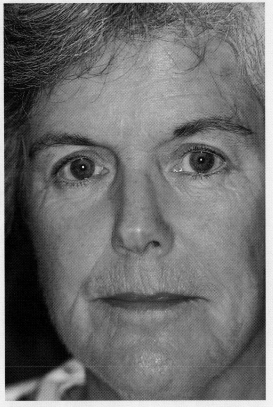

Case 8.2B After

*From Kauvar AB, Geronemus RG. Laser therapy of cutaneous vascular lesions. *Operative Techniques Otolaryngol Head Neck Surg* 1994; Vol. 5:250–258.

REFERENCES

1. Merlen JF. Red telangiectasias, blue telangiectasias. *Soc Franc Phlebol* 1970;22:167–74.
2. Bean WB. *Vascular spiders and related lesions of the skin.* Springfield: Thomas, 1958.
3. Alderson MR. Spider naevi—their incidence in healthy school children. *Arch Dis Child* 1963;38:286–8.
4. Goldman MP, Fitzpatrick RE. Pulsed dye laser treatment of leg telangiectasia: with and without simultaneous sclerotherapy. *J Dermatol Surg Oncol* 1990;16:338–44.
5. Geronemus R. Treatment of spider telangiectasias in children using the flashlamp-pumped pulsed dye laser. *Pediatr Dermatol* 1991;8:61–3.
6. Goldman MP, Bennett RG. Treatment of telangiectasia: a review. *J Am Acad Dermatol* 1987;17:167–82.
7. Redisch W, Pelzer RH. Localized vascular dilatations of the human skin: capillary microscopy and related studies. *Am Heart J* 1949;37:106–14.
8. Bodian EL. Techniques of sclerotherapy for sunburst venous blemishes. *J Dermatol Surg Oncol* 1985;11:696–704.
9. Faria JL, Moraes IN. Histopathology of the telangiectasias associated with varicose veins. *Dermatologica* 1963;127:321–9.
10. Mullikan JB, Young AE. *Vascular birthmarks. Hemangiomas and malformations.* Philadelphia: Saunders, 1988.
11. Wenzl JE, Burgert EO. The spider nevus in infancy and childhood. *Pediatrics* 1964;33:227–32.
12. McGrae JD, Winkelmann RK. Generalized essential telangiectasia: report of a clinical and histochemical study of 13 patients with acquired cutaneous lesions. *JAMA* 1963;185:909.
13. Rosenwasser TA, Eisen AZ. Scleroderma. In: Fitzpatrick TB, Eisen AZ, Wolff K, et al., eds. *Dermatology in general medicine.* New York: McGraw-Hill, 1993;2156–67.
14. Moy JA. Cutaneous manifestations of drug abuse. In: Fitzpatrick TB, Eisen AZ, Wolff K, et al., eds. *Dermatology in general medicine.* New York: McGraw-Hill, 1993;1807–12.
15. Freinkel RK. Cutaneous manifestations of endocrine diseases. In: Fitzpatrick TB, Eisen AZ, Wolff K, et al., eds. *Dermatology in general medicine.* New York: McGraw-Hill, 1993;2113–31.
16. Stoughton RB, Corness RC. Corticosteroids. In: Fitzpatrick TB, Eisen AZ, Wolff K, et al., eds. *Dermatology in general medicine.* New York: McGraw-Hill, 1993;2846–50.
17. Kligman AM, Kligman LH. Photoaging. In: Fitzpatrick TB, Eisen AZ, Wolff K, et al., eds. *Dermatology in general medicine.* New York: McGraw-Hill, 1993;2972–9.
18. Sobye P. Aetiology and pathogenesis of rosacea. *Acta Derm Venereol (Stockh)* 1950;30:137–58.
19. Marks R. Concepts in the pathogenesis of rosacea. *Br J Dermatol* 1968;80:170–7.
20. Thulesius O. Physiologic observations on causes of varicose veins. In: Bergen JJ, Goldman MP, eds. *Varicose veins and telangiectasias.*

Diagnosis and treatment. St Louis: Quality Medical Publishing, 1993;3–11.

21. Noe JM, Finley J, Rosen S, Arndt KA. Postrhinoplasty "red nose": differential diagnosis and treatment by laser. *Plast Reconstr Surg* 1981;67:661–4.

22. Goslen JB. Wound healing for the dermatologic surgeon. *J Dermatol Surg Oncol* 1988;14:959–72.

23. Folkman J, Klagsbrun M. Angiogenic factors. *Science* 1987;235:442–7.

24. Goldman MP, Weiss RA, Brody HJ, Coleman WP, Fitzpatrick RE. Treatment of facial telangiectasia with sclerotherapy, laser surgery, and/or electrodesiccation: a review. *J Dermatol Surg Oncol* 1993;19:889–906.

25. Wilkin JK. Flushing reactions. In: Rook AJ, Maibach HI, eds. *Recent advances in dermatology,* No. 6. New York: Churchill-Livingstone, 1983;157–87.

26. Weiss RA, Weiss MA. Resolution of pain associated with varicose and telangiectatic leg veins after compression sclerotherapy. *J Dermatol Surg Oncol* 1990;16:333–6.

27. Kirsch N. Telangiectasia and electrolysis [letter]. *J Dermatol Surg Oncol* 1984;10:9–10.

28. Recoules-Arche J. Electrocoagulation. *Phlebologie* 1966;33:885.

29. Thibault PK. Treatment of telangiectasias. In: Bergen JJ, Goldman MP, eds. *Varicose veins and telangiectasias. Diagnosis and treatment.* St Louis: Quality Medical Publishing, 1993;373–88.

30. Goldman MP, Kaplan RP, Duffy DM. Postsclerotherapy hyperpigmentation: a histologic evaluation. *J Dermatol Surg Oncol* 1987;13:547–50.

31. Duffy DM. Small vessel sclerotherapy: an overview. In: Callen JP, Dahl MV, Golitz LE, et al., eds. *Advances in dermatology,* vol 3. Chicago: Year Book, 1988;221–42.

32. Alster TS, Kohn SR. Dermatologic lasers: three decades of progress. *Int J Dermatol* 1992;31:601–10.

33. Geronemus RG. Argon laser for the treatment of cutaneous lesions. *Clin Dermatol,* 1995;13:55–58.

34. Dover JS, Arndt KA, Geronemus RG, et al. Understanding lasers. In: *Illustrated cutaneous laser surgery: a practitioner's guide.* Norwalk CT: Appleton & Lange, 1990;1–19.

35. Garden JM, Geronemus RG. Dermatologic laser surgery. *J Dermatol Surg Oncol* 1990;16:156.

36. Apfelberg DB, Maser MR, Lash H. Expanded role of the argon laser in plastic surgery. *J Dermatol Surg Oncol* 1983;9:145–9.

37. Apfelberg DB, Maser MR, Lash H, et al. The argon laser for cutaneous lesions. *JAMA* 1981;245:2073–5.

38. Goldman MP, Fitzpatrick RE. Treatment of cutaneous vascular lesions. In: Goldman MP, Fitzpatrick RE, eds. Cutaneous laser surgery: the art and science of selective photothermolysis. St Louis: Mosby, 1994;19–105.

39. Key D. Argon-pumped tunable dye laser for the treatment of cutaneous lesions. *Clin Dermatol,* 1995;13:59–61.

40. Glassberg E, Walker K, Lask GP. Lasers in dermatology. In: Lask GP, et al., eds. *Principles and techniques of cutaneous surgery,* McGraw Hill 1995 (In press).

108

41. Ofrenstein A, Nelson SJ. Treatment of facial vascular lesions with a 100 micron spot 577 nm pulsed continuous wave dye laser. *Ann Plast Surg* 1989;23:310–6.

42. Mordon S, Beacco C, Rotteleur G, Brunstaud JM. Relation between skin surface temperature and minimal blanching during argon, Nd:YAG, and cw dye 585 laser therapy of port-wine stains. *Laser Surg Med* 1993;13:124–6.

43. Apfelberg DB, Smoller B. Preliminary analysis of histological results of hexascan device with continuous tunable dye laser at 514 (argon) and 577 nm (yellow). *Laser Surg Med* 1993;13:106–12.

44. McDaniel DH. Cutaneous vascular disorders: advances in laser treatments. *Cutis* 1990;45:339–59.

45. McDaniel DH. Clinical applications of lasers for skin disorders: comparisons and contrasts. *Skinlaser Today* 1992;5–13.

46. Keller GS. Use of the KTP laser in cosmetic surgery. *Am J Cosmetic Surg* 1992;9:177–80.

47. Goldman L. New developments with the heavy metal vapor lasers for the dermatologist. *J Dermatol Surg Oncol* 1987;13:163.

48. Schliftman AB, Brauner G. The comparative tissue effects of copper vapor laser (578 nm) on vascular lesions [abstract]. *Laser Surg Med* 1988;8:188.

49. Waner M, Dinehart S, Wilson M, Flock S. A comparison of copper vapor and flashlamp-pumped dye lasers in treatment of facial telangiectasia. *J Dermatol Surg Oncol* 1993;19:992–8.

50. Dinehart S, Waner M, Flock S. The copper vapor laser for treatment of cutaneous vascular and pigmented lesions. *J Dermatol Surg Oncol* 1993;19:370–5.

51. Hruza GJ, Geronemus RG, Dover JS, Arndt KA. Lasers in dermatology—1993. *Arch Dermatol* 1993;129:1026–35.

52. Anderson RR, Parish JA. Microvasculature can be selectively damaged using dye lasers: a basic theory and experimental evidence in human skin. *Lasers Surg Med* 1981;1:263–76.

53. Garden JM, Tan OT, Kerschmann R, et al. Effect of dye laser pulse duration on selective cutaneous vascular injury. *J Invest Dermatol* 1986;87:653–7.

54. Goldman MP, Fitzpatrick RE, Ruiz-Esparza J. Treatment of spider telangiectasia in children. *Contemp Pediatr* 1993;10:16.

55. Fitzpatrick RE, Goldman MP. Treatment of facial telangiectasia with the flashlamp-pumped dye laser. *Lasers Surg Med Suppl* 1991;3:70.

56. Gonzalez E, Gange RW, Momtaz K. Treatment of telangiectasias and other benign vascular lesions with the 577 nm pulsed dye laser. *J Am Acad Dermatol* 1992;27:220–4.

57. Lowe NJ, Behr KL, Fitzpatrick R, Goldman M, Ruiz-Esparza J. Flashlamp-pumped dye laser for rosacea-associated telangiectasia and erythema. *J Dermatol Surg Oncol* 1991;17:522–5.

58. Potozkin JR, Geronemus RG. Treatment of poikilodermatous component of the Rothmund–Thomson syndrome with the flashlamp-pumped pulsed dye laser: a case report. *Pediatr Dermatol* 1991;8:162–5.

59. Alster TS, Wilson F. Treatment of focal dermal hypoplasia (Goltz syndrome) with the 585 nm flashlamp-pumped pulsed dye laser. *Arch Dermatol* 1995;131:143–4

60. Civatte A. Poikilodermie reticulae pigmentaire du visage et du colline. *Ann Dermatol Syph* 1923;6:605.

61. Geronemus RG. Poikiloderma of Civatte [letter]. *Arch Dermatol* 1990;126:547–8.

62. Tan OT, Kurban AK. Noncongenital benign cutaneous vascular lesions: pulse dye laser treatment. In: Tan OT, ed. *Management and treatment of benign cutaneous vascular lesions.* Philadelphia: Lea & Febiger, 1992.

63. Polla LL, Tan OT, Garden JM, et al. Tunable dye laser for the treatment of benign cutaneous vascular ectasia. *Dermatologica* 1987;174:11–7.

64. Broska P, Martinho E, Goodman M. Comparisons of the argon tunable dye laser with the flashlamp pulsed dye laser in treatment of facial telangiectasia. *J Dermatol Surg Oncol* 1994;20:749–54.

9

LASER TREATMENT OF TATTOOS AND PIGMENTED LESIONS

Suzanne L. Kilmer, M.D.

Tina S. Alster, M.D.

9.1 INTRODUCTION

Physicians are often consulted to remove cosmetically disfiguring tattoos and pigmented lesions. Until the most recent developments in laser technology, however, these lesions could not be eradicated without significant sequelae, such as scarring and dyspigmentation. This chapter will discuss and compare the scope of lasers currently available to treat these popular and common lesions.

9.2 TATTOOS

Tattoos are the visible result of exogenous material implanted in the dermis, usually by tattoo artists, cosmetologists, or a traumatic event. The fascination with decorative tattoos continues, with over 10 million people in the United States sporting at least one tattoo. Long considered permanent, tattoos are also placed for identification purposes (prisoners of war, gang members) or to mark a location, as in radiation ports, for medicinal purposes. Cosmetic tattoos in which black, red, or brown pigments are tattooed to mimic eye, lip, or eyebrow liner, have also become increasingly popular. In addition, flesh-toned pigments have been injected within vascular and

Cosmetic Laser Surgery, Edited by Alster, M.D. and Apfelberg, M.D.
ISBN 0471-12242-4 © 1996 Wiley-Liss, Inc.

112

pigmented birthmarks, as well as over undesired tattoos, for camouflaging purposes. Finally, traumatic tattoos arise from the undesired implantation of graphite, asphalt, or gunpowder into the skin with visible consequences.

A long history and existence prior to regulatory agencies have enabled tattooing to remain an unlicensed, yet invasive, procedure for many years. A needle or tattoo gun is used to introduce ink into the dermis (with potential transmission of hepatitis or HIV by contaminated needles) where it remains free until engulfed by macrophages, the predominant responding phagocyte. Ink particles have been found in draining lymph nodes prior to any attempt at tattoo removal, suggesting lymphatic drainage as one mode of ink dispersement. The majority of ink particles are too large to be carried away, however, accounting for the permanence of tattooed lesions.

In most cases, tattoos maintain their varied colors and designs as originally placed, rarely inciting any tissue reaction, although many tattoos fade and become less distinct with time. In a few individuals, however, some inks may incite an allergic response with an erythematous, indurated region in part or all of the tattoo. This is most frequently seen with red ink (1–5), in response to the mercuric sulfide base of the red pigment, but can also be elicited by blue (cobalt) (6), green (chromium) (7), or yellow (cadmium) (8) inks. Rarely, a systemic response may even be triggered (9).

9.3 PIGMENTED LESIONS

Pigmented cutaneous lesions result from the presence of melanin-containing cells (melanocytes) in the epidermis and/or dermis. Superficial pigmented lesions, such as café-au-lait spots and solar lentigines, usually contain an increased number of melanocytes at the basal layer of the epidermis (10–12). More deeply pigmented lesions, such as nevus of Ota and other congenital nevi, contain melanocytes in the papillary and reticular dermis (13).

Solar lentigines (or age spots) are always a result of excessive ultraviolet exposure and are seen in the majority of the adult population. Sun-exposed areas, such as the face, dorsal hands, and anterior chest, are commonly involved. Congenital birthmarks, such as café-au-lait spots and nevi of Ota, are found in upward of 10% of the population. They frequently present for treatment due to their obvious cosmetic disfigurement.

9.4 LASER TREATMENT

9.4.1 Background
Historically, traditional modalities employed to remove tattoos and pigmented lesions had centered around tissue removal or destruction in the area of ink or pigment deposition. Dermabrasion or sal-

113

abrasion with or without the addition of chemicals (14–18), cryosurgery (19), surgical excision (20–24), and electrosurgery (25,26) have all been effective in removing tattoo ink and cutaneous pigment; however, the resultant scar or dyspigmentation was often as undesirable as the original lesion.

Laser treatment of cutaneous lesions was first pioneered by Leon Goldman in the 1960s, when he and others used a ruby laser to treat pigmented lesions and tattoos (27–29). Unfortunately, technical difficulties curtailed research using the ruby laser for many years. The carbon dioxide laser was subsequently used to treat a variety of lesions through vaporization of the superficial cutaneous layers (30–33). Scarring, due to thermal denaturation of collagen, was a significant drawback seen with the use of the carbon dioxide laser, which was only minimally improved with the later use of the argon laser (34–37).

Selective photothermolysis, the concept of producing preferential injury to pigment-containing structures using brief, selectively absorbed laser pulses (38), revolutionized the use of laser treatment for a variety of cutaneous lesions. By using a wavelength that is selectively absorbed by the target and a pulse duration shorter than or equal to the thermal relaxation time of the desired microscopic structure, damage could effectively be contained within the targeted tissue (39). Using these principles, endogenous chromophores (hemoglobin, melanin), as well as exogenous chromophores (tattoo ink, graphite), can be targeted while leaving the adjacent collagen intact, thereby minimizing the potential for scarring.

Ultrashort pulse durations (nanoseconds, ns) seen in Q-switched (QS) laser systems are critical for the treatment of tattoos and pigmented lesions. In the case of tattoos, the high energy delivered leads to extremely high temperatures over a very short time period, resulting in rapid thermal expansion of ink particles with subsequent shattering. The ultimate fate of laser-irradiated tattoo ink is not well understood. Ink removal is inhibited by the large particle size, as well as by engulfment by immobile macrophages. The lymph system presumably plays a significant role in clearing the pigment after shattering of the particles, which frees them from macrophage entrapment. Changes in optical properties also play a role in the apparent improvement seen. Six weeks following QS laser irradiation, residual dermal tattoo ink appears markedly smaller, less dense, and paler in color (40,41). The epidermis is preserved with negligible dermal fibrosis, which is in contrast to the histology seen following argon laser treatment (42).

In the treatment of pigmented lesions, melanosomal alterations have been shown to be qualitatively similar at a wide range of wavelengths but differ in threshold dose and depth of penetration into the dermis. Shorter wavelengths of light require less energy to damage the epidermal pigment cell, whereas longer wavelengths are capable of deeper (dermal) penetration. Specificity of injury to epidermal pigment has been shown to be greatest at 504 nm (43), utilizing a pulse duration that corresponds to the 1-microsecond (μs)

114

thermal relaxation time of the targeted melanosome (44–46). Dermal pigment, on the other hand, is most effectively treated with lasers at longer wavelengths and short pulse durations, such as the QSRL, QS Nd:YAG, and QS alexandrite lasers, due to their capacity for deeper tissue penetration (47–49). Pigment cells are selectively destroyed, presumably as a result of either extreme temperature gradients created within melanosomes or from shock-wave/cavitation damage that results from rapid thermal expansion (50).

Thus with the advent of QS lasers, progression was made from gross tissue destruction to selective removal of tattoo ink and epidermal and dermal pigment without scarring. The QS ruby laser at 694 nm (QSRL) was the first laser to accomplish this until the more recent additions of the QS neodymium:yttrium aluminum garnet laser at 532 and 1064 nm (Nd:YAG), QS alexandrite laser at 755 nm, and pigmented lesion dye laser (PLDL) at 510 nm.

Successful removal of tattoos using the QSRL was reported in 1983 by Reid et al. (51) with subsequent reports confirming the efficacy and excellent cosmetic outcome achieved (52–54). The inability of the QSRL to treat most red inks and its strong affinity for melanin (commonly leading to hypopigmentation) were limiting factors when treating darker skin tones and professional tattoos (one-third of which contain red tattoo ink). The Nd:YAG laser at 1064 nm was shown to have less melanin absorption and deeper tissue penetration (55–57). In addition, the introduction of a frequency-doubling crystal with the 1064-nm Nd:YAG produced 532-nm green light, which is well absorbed by red ink. The QS alexandrite laser at 755 nm is also effective in the treatment of black, blue, and green inks (58–60). Its frequent association with the 510-nm pulsed dye laser permits treatment of red ink as well (59). All the QS systems have been shown to be effective in eliminating pigmented cutaneous lesions. While the frequency-doubled Nd:YAG laser (532 nm) and PLDL (510 nm) are effective in treating only epidermal pigment as a result of superficial penetration (61–65), the QS ruby, Nd:YAG, and QS alexandrite lasers are able to penetrate and eliminate deeper pigment more readily (66–73).

9.4.2 General Laser Treatment Principles

Many treatment principles are common to all of the QS laser systems. While the different wavelengths account for variations in absorption and efficacy for different tattoo colors and pigmented lesions, all the QS laser systems are somewhat painful, require multiple treatment sessions, and have similar risks for hyperpigmentation and textural changes. Further elaboration on these issues follows.

Unlike with prior carbon dioxide and argon laser treatment, many patients are able to tolerate QS lasers without anesthesia. The sensation most often described is that of a snap of a rubber band or of bacon grease hitting the skin. A few laser pulses may be given to assess the patient's tolerance to treatment. If anesthesia is desired, it

TABLE 9.1 Response of Different Tattoo Ink Colors to Current QS Lasers

TATTOO INK	RUBY (694 nm)	ALEXANDRITE (755 nm)	Nd:YAG (1064 nm)	Nd:YAG/2 (532 nm)	PLDL (510 nm)
Blue/black	+++	+++	+++	−	−
Green	++	++	+/−	−	−
Red	−	−	−	+	+
Orange	−	−	−	+	+
Flesh/white	black	black	black	black	black

can be administered locally with 1–2% lidocaine or topically using EMLA (eutectic mixture of lidocaine and prilocaine) or 30–40% lidocaine in a water-miscible base (i.e., acid mantle or velvachol) under occlusion for 30–90 minutes (74).

Given the multitude of colored inks available and the varying response to treatment, it is difficult to predict how many laser treatments are needed to clear a tattoo; however, use of a wavelength well absorbed by the tattoo ink enhances the ability to treat that particular color (Table 9.1). In general, amateur tattoos are easier to clear than professional tattoos, presumably due to the type and amount of ink contained in the tattoo (professional tattoos have large amounts of metallo-organic dyes versus amateur tattoos, which have smaller amounts of carbon-based ink). In addition, older tattoos fare better than recently placed tattoos, as the body slowly disperses ink over time.

Red, brown, flesh-toned, and white inks, which are commonly seen in cosmetic tattoos of the lips, eyebrows, and eyelids, have been noted to turn slate-gray or black after QS laser treatment (75) as a result of the iron oxide- or titanium oxide-based pigments in these tattoo colors (Figure 9.1). It is not currently possible to predict

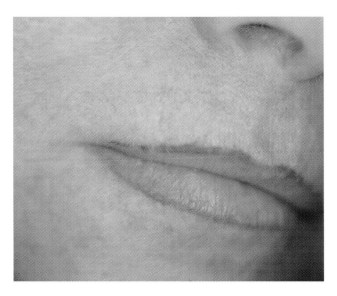

FIGURE 9.1 35-year-old woman with maroon lip liner tattoo placed 1 year prior to presentation. Test area using QS Nd:YAG laser at 532 nm, 2.0 J/cm^2, 3-mm spot size showed immediate darkening of tattoo. Subsequent retreatment of darkened tattoo with QS Nd:YAG at 1064 nm, 6.0 J/cm^2, and 3-mm spot size showed eventual tattoo clearing.

115

which inks will darken or, in those cases that have darkened following QS laser irradiation, which ones will lighten with further laser treatments.

The high-energy, ultrashort QS laser pulses can cause epidermal debris for which a clear protective barrier (i.e., Vigilon), should be used to limit tissue splatter during treatment. Conical devices to contain the debris during treatment have been developed. Wound care following treatment with any one of the QS laser systems is similar and consists of application of antibiotic ointment and a clean nonstick bandage following gentle cleansing with mild soap and water once or twice daily until all crusting resolves (usually 10–14 days).

Treatment protocols, side effects, and follow-up for each laser system are reviewed separately below. While specific treatment parameters are provided, it is important to use them only as guidelines and to evaluate each patient's skin type and lesional response individually.

9.4.3 Q-Switched Ruby Laser (694 nm)

The red light emitted by the ruby laser is well absorbed by green and black tattoo inks. Absorption by melanin is also fairly strong, which is the reason why this laser is helpful for removing pigmented lesions. Unfortunately, the melanin selectivity hinders treatment of darker skin tones and may lead to increased hypopigmentation following treatment of tattoos.

The latest QSRL models have pulse durations of 25 ns, spot sizes of 5.0–6.5 mm, and a pulse delivery rate of 1 hertz (Hz). Treatment is usually initiated at a fluence of 6–8 Joules/cm^2 (J/cm^2). The aim is to achieve immediate whitening within the tattoo or pigmented lesion without perforation of the skin. If perforation (tissue splatter or bleeding) occurs, the fluence should be reduced. The entire area can be treated in one sitting. With subsequent treatment sessions, the fluence may need to be increased to remove the remaining ink or pigment.

Blue-black and green tattoo pigments are the most responsive to the QSRL. In general, amateur tattoos require four to six treatment sessions and professional tattoos require six to ten sessions (51–54). Many more sessions may be needed to achieve the desired clinical clearing in heavily tattooed lesions.

Epidermal pigmented lesions such as solar lentigines clear easily within one to two QSRL treatments, whereas café-au-lait macules require three or four treatments at 5.0–6.0 J/cm^2. Dermal melanocytic lesions, such as nevus of Ota, require an average of four to six QSRL treatments using similar parameters for removal (68–71).

Complications following QSRL treatment are often associated with excessive melanin absorption, commonly leading to transient hypopigmentation and, rarely, to permanent depigmentation

CASE 9.2 FIFTEEN-YEAR-OLD MULTICOLORED PROFESSIONAL TATTOO

A 40-year-old woman with multicolored professional tattoo on the shoulder, which was placed 15 years prior to presentation (Case Figure 9.2A). Other decorative tattoos were present on the ankles. No prior treatment had been received.

Anesthesia: None.

Procedure: Twelve Q-switched alexandrite laser treatments at an average fluence of 7.0 J/cm^2 were delivered over the entire tattoo at 8-week intervals. Three PLDL (510-nm) treatments at 3.0 J/cm^2 were used to eliminate the red tattoo pigment.

Postoperative Care: Twice daily cleansing with mild soap and water followed by application of bacitracin ointment and nonstick bandage for 10–14 days.

Postoperative Results: Eight weeks following the final alexandrite laser treatment, the tattoo was completely eliminated without evidence of textural change, scarring, or pigmentary alteration (Case Figure 9.2B).

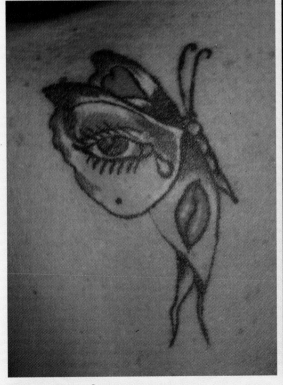

Case 9.2A Before   Case 9.2B After

CASE 9.3 SOLAR LENTIGINES

A 29-year-old woman with solar lentigines of the anterior chest present since her teenage years (Case Figure 9.3A). Patient admitted to frequent suntanning and had been a regular user of tanning salons in the winter months. She had no family or personal history of skin cancer or atypical moles.

Anesthesia: None.

Procedure: One frequency-doubled QS Nd:YAG (532 nm, 5 ns, 3 mm spot, 10 Hz) treatment session at 2.0 J/cm.^{2} (Solar lentigines can also be treated with QS ruby 510 nm pulsed dye lasers.)

Postoperative Care: Daily rinse with mild soap and water followed by application of antibiotic ointment until all crusting cleared (7–10 days).

Postoperative Results: Total clearing of lesions with normal tanning of laser-treated skin (Case Figure 9.3B).

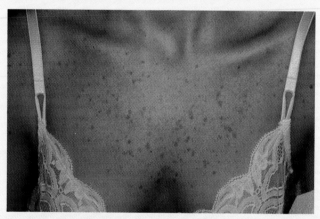

Case 9.3A Before

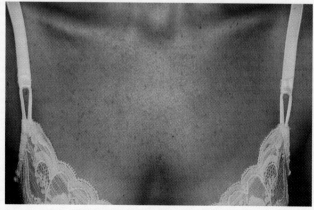

Case 9.3B After

CASE 9.4 CAFÉ-AU-LAIT BIRTHMARK

An 8-year-old boy with a café-au-lait birthmark involving his left cheek (Case Figure 9.4A). The lesion had grown commensurate with his body growth and no changes in color had been noted with advancing age. No prior treatment had been obtained.

Anesthesia: A 30% lidocaine cream in velvachol cream base occluded with Tegederm for 30 minutes.

Procedure: Eight PLDL (510 nm, 300 ns) laser sessions at 8–10-week intervals at fluences ranging from 2.0 to 3.0 J/cm^2 with a 5-mm spot size. (Café-au-lait birthmarks can also be treated with QS ruby and QS Nd:YAG lasers.)

Postoperative Care: Daily cleansing with mild soap and water followed by application of antibiotic ointment and a nonstick bandage. Strict sunscreen use was required between laser sessions.

Postoperative Results: Complete elimination of café-au-lait pigment was noted 2 months following the eighth laser treatment (Case Figure 9.4B). Note the normal freckling of skin overlying the lesion. No recurrence of the lesion was noted at 1 year following the last laser treatment.

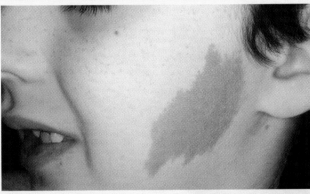

Case 9.4A Before

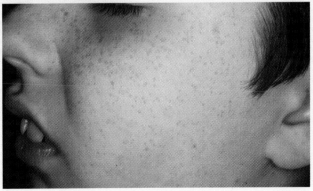

Case 9.4B After

CASE 9.5 NEVUS OF OTA

An 18-year-old man with nevus of Ota involving his right cheek and temple (Case Figure 9.5A). Lesion was apparent at birth but had become darker with advancing age.

Anesthesia: None.

Procedure: Five Q-switched alexandrite (755 nm, 100 ns, 1 Hz)* laser treatments at a mean fluence of 6.5 J/cm^2 every 8–12 weeks. Entire lesion was treated with adjacent, nonoverlapping laser pulses with a characteristic tissue whitening observed with laser impact. No tissue debris or blood splatter was encountered.

Postoperative Care: Twice daily cleansing with mild soap and water followed by application of antibiotic ointment and nonstick bandage for 1–2 weeks.

Postoperative Results: Total resolution of lesion noted at 3 months following fifth and final laser treatment (Case Figure 9.5B). One-year follow-up has revealed no lesional recurrence.

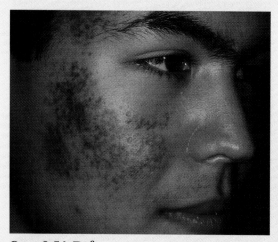

Case 9.5A Before

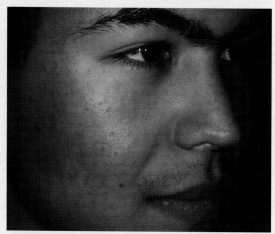

Case 9.5B After

*The Q-switched ruby or Nd:YAG laser could also have been used in this case with similar results.

REFERENCES

1. Roenigk HH. Tattooing: history, technics, complications, removal. *Cleve Clin Q* 1971;38:181–6.
2. Lever WP, Lever GS. Foreign body reactions. In: *Histopathology of the skin*. Philadelphia: Lippincott, 1983;221–6.
3. Ackerman BA. Nodular and diffuse dermatitis. In: *Histologic diagnosis of inflammatory skin diseases*. Philadelphia: Lea & Febiger, 1978;436–42.
4. Madden JF. Reactions in tattoos. *Arch Dermatol Syph* 1939;40:256–62.
5. Abel EA, Silberberg I, Queen D. Studies of chronic inflammation in a red tattoo by electron microscopy and histochemistry. *Acta Derm Venereol (Stockh)* 1972;54:453–61.
6. Bjornberg A. Allergic reaction to cobalt in light blue tattoo markings. *Acta Derm Venereol (Stockh)* 1961;41:259–63.
7. Loewenthal LA. Reactions in green tattoos. *Arch Dermatol* 1973;107:101–3.
8. Bjornberg A. Reactions to light in yellow tattoos from cadmium sulfide. *Arch Dermatol* 1963;88:267.
9. Novy FG. A generalized mercurial (cinnabar) reaction following tattooing. *Arch Dermatol* 1944;49:172.
10. Fulk C. Primary disorders of hyperpigmentation. *J Am Acad Dermatol* 1984;10:1–16.
11. Johnson BL, Charneco DR. Cafe au lait spots in neurofibromatosis and in normal individuals. *Arch Dermatol* 1970;102:442–6.
12. Takahashi M, Studies on café-au-lait spots in neurofibromatosis and pigmented macules of nevus spilus. *Tokohu J Exp Med* 1976;18:225–73.
13. Lever WF, Schaumburg-Lever G. *Histopathology of the Skin.* Philadelphia: JB Lippincott Co. pp. 699–700.
14. Scutt RW. The chemical removal of tattoos. *Br J Plast Surg* 1972;25:189–94.
15. Manchester GH. Removal of commercial tattoos by abrasion with table salt. *Plast Reconstr Surg* 1974;53:517–21.
16. Crittenden FM. Salabrasion: removal of tattoos by superficial abrasion with table salt. *Cutis* 1971;7:295–300.
17. Clabaugh W. Removal of tattoos by superficial dermabrasion. *Arch Dermatol* 1968;98:515–21.
18. Koerber WA, Price NM. Salabrasion of tattoos. *Arch Dermatol* 1978;114:884–8.
19. Dvir E, Hirshowitz B. Tattoo removal by cryosurgery. *Plast Reconstr Surg* 1980;66:373–8.
20. Buncke HR Jr, Conway H. Surgery of decorative and traumatic tattoos. *Plast Reconst Surg* 1957;20:67–77.
21. Bailey BN. Treatment of tattoos. *Plast Reconstr Surg* 1967;10:361–71.
22. Fujimori Y. Treatment of nevus of Ota and nevus spilus. In: *Skin surface surgery*. Tokyo: Kokuseido, 1990;181–8.
23. Kobayashi T. Microsurgical treatment of nevus of Ota. *J Dermatol Surg Oncol* 1991;17:936–41.

125

24. Cosman B, Apfelberg DB, Druker D. An effective cosmetic treatment for Ota's nevus. *Ann Plast Surg* 1989;22:36–42.

25. Groot DW, Arlette JP, Johnston PA. Comparison of the infrared coagulator and the carbon dioxide laser in the removal of decorative tattoos. *J Am Acad Dermatol* 1986;15:518–22.

26. Colver GB, Cherry GW, Dawber RPR, Ryan TJ. Tattoo removal using infrared coagulation. *Br J Dermatol* 1985;112:481–5.

27. Goldman L, Hornby P, Meyer R. Radiation from a Q-switched laser with a total output of 10 megawatts on a tattoo of a man. *J Invest Dermatol* 1965;44:69.

28. Goldman L, Rockwell RJ, Meyer R, et al. Laser treatment of tattoos: a preliminary survey of three years clinical experience. *JAMA* 1967;201:163–6.

29. Yules RB, Laub DR, Honey R, et al. The effect of Q-switched ruby laser radiation on dermal tattoo pigment in man. *Arch Surg* 1967;95:179–80.

30. Bailin PL, Ratz JR, Levine HL. Removal of tattoos by CO_2 laser. *J Dermatol Surg Oncol* 1980;6:997–1001.

31. Reid R, Muller S. Tattoo removal by CO_2 laser dermabrasion. *Plast Reconstr Surg* 1980;65:717–21.

32. Fitzpatrick RE, Ruiz-Esparza JN, Goldman MP. The depth of thermal necrosis using the CO_2 laser: a comparison of the superpulsed mode and conventional modes. *J Dermatol Surg Oncol* 1991;17:340–4.

33. Ruiz-Esparza J, Goldman MP, Fitzpatrick RE. Tattoo removal with minimal scarring: the chemo-laser technique. *J Dermatol Surg Oncol* 1989;14:1372–6.

34. Apfelberg DB, Maser MR, Lash H, et al. Comparison of the argon and carbon dioxide laser treatment of decorative tattoos: a preliminary report. *Ann Plast Surg* 1985;14:6–15.

35. Apfelberg DB, Maser MR, Lash H, Rivers J. The argon laser for cutaneous lesions. *JAMA* 1981;245:2073–6.

36. Oshiro T, Maruyama Y. The ruby and argon lasers in the treatment of naevi. *Ann Acad Med Singapore* 1983;12:388–91.

37. Trelles MA, Verkruysse W, Pickering JW, et al. Monoline argon laser (514 nm) treatment of benign pigmented lesions with long pulse lengths. *J Photochem Photobiol* 1992;16:357–60.

38. Anderson RR, Parrish JA. Selective photothermolysis: precise microsurgery by selective absorption of pulsed irradiation. *Science* 1983;220:524–7.

39. Anderson RR, Parrish JA. Microvasculature can be selectively damaged using dye lasers: a basic theory and experimental evidence in human skin. *Lasers Surg Med* 1981;1:263–7.

40. Taylor CR, Anderson RR, Gange W, et al. Light and electron microscopic analysis of tattoos by Q-switched ruby laser. *J Invest Dermatol* 1991;97:131–6.

41. Kilmer SL, Lee MS, Grevelink JM, et al. The Q-switched Nd:YAG laser (1064 nm) effectively treats tattoos: a controlled, dose–response study. *Arch Dermatol* 1993;129:971–8.

42. Diette KM, Bronstein BR, Parrish JA. Histologic comparison of argon and tunable dye lasers in the treatment of tattoos. *J Invest Dermatol* 1985;85:368–42.

43. Sherwood KA, Murray S, Kurban AK, Tan OT. Effect of wavelength on

SAMPLE PATIENT AND PRACTICE ANNOUNCEMENT LETTER II

Dear Patient:

The _____ Laser Center is proud to announce the addition of a new laser to our facility. The _____ laser offers the newest state-of-the-art laser technology. With this laser, we are able to treat {red spots such as spider veins, angiomas, and port-wine stains, brown spots such as sun spots, café-au-lait birthmarks, and moles, tattoos, scars, wrinkles, (other)] without scarring.

Treatment can usually be accomplished in a short office visit (30 minutes) without general anesthesia. Sometimes a numbing cream or local anesthetic is used to lessen the "snapping" sensation of the laser. Although several treatments may be required, the final results show marked lightening or total removal of these blemishes without significant skin changes, such as scarring.

If you have an unwanted skin blemish that you would like treated, please call our office to arrange for a consultation. At that time, we would be happy to discuss the procedure, treatment scheduling, and anticipated cost with you.

Sincerely,

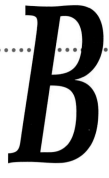

APPENDIX
PATIENT INFORMATION
AND
CONSENT FORMS

136 SAMPLE INFORMATION AND CONSENT FORM FOR LASER RESURFACING

The carbon dioxide laser has been a popular surgeon's tool over the past several years, but its use has been limited due to the risk of scarring and pigmentary changes resulting from the deep thermal damage (or heat buildup) it produces in the skin. The Ultrapulse laser has eliminated this problem with the development of a high-energy, short-pulse waveform, which can limit the thermal impact to the most superficial portion (or outer layer) of the skin.

When the skin is treated with the Ultrapulse laser, a clean, layer-by-layer vaporization of the skin occurs. The undesired skin literally evaporates due to the high water content of the epidermis. The laser is therefore best-suited for those skin conditions that are superficial in nature, such as fine lines and wrinkles, blotchiness (or dark and light patches), keratoses (pre-cancers), scaling, and mild acne scarring. The skin in these conditions is "resurfaced" or "rejuvenated" by the vaporizing action of the laser.

The procedure is quick, bloodless, and does not require general anesthesia. The healing process takes place over 1 to 2 weeks, leaving a pink, smoother, "new" skin. Because the Ultrapulse laser is so precise, the risk of scarring or other complications (such as infection) is minimized.

* * * * *

I, _____, consent to laser resurfacing of the skin on my face. I understand that, even in the most experienced surgeon's hands, the following complications may rarely occur:

1. Skin depression or scarring
2. Dyspigmentation (skin lightening or darkening)
3. Infection
4. Persistent facial redness
5. Demarcation lines or patches
6. Incomplete removal of damaged skin, scars, or wrinkles
7. Cold sores
8. Swelling
9. Allergy to antibiotic ointment

I authorize the taking of photographs. All my questions regarding the laser treatment and postoperative care have been answered to my satisfaction.

_____   _____

Patient signature (Printed name)   Date

_____

Witness

SAMPLE PATIENT INFORMATION AND CONSENT FORM FOR LASER TREATMENT OF SCARS

137

A scar can develop in the skin anytime there is injury or trauma to the skin. Sometimes a more severe type of scar will develop that may be red and raised (hypertrophic) or grow into a large nodule that extends beyond the margins of the original wound (keloid). Hypertrophic scars and keloids affect an estimated 4.5% to 16% of the population and have been difficult to treat in the past because they have a tendency to return.

Laser surgery using a new pulsed laser has been shown to improve these scars by reducing their redness and height, altering the skin texture to one that is more normal, improving pliability (softness), and eliminating symptoms, such as burning or itching. As few as one or two laser treatments are usually necessary; however, with thicker scars, several more sessions may be needed to achieve the desired amount of scar improvement. The treatments are delivered every 6 to 8 weeks to allow adequate time for proper healing of the skin. Immediately after treatment, the scar will appear bruised. The deep purple or black color will last approximately 1 to 2 weeks, after which time, the scar will begin appearing less red and will become flatter and softer. You may notice some itching during the healing phase. In patients with darker skin tones, hyperpigmentation (or a brownish skin discoloration) within the laser-treated scar may develop, which will eventually disappear. When used properly, the pulsed laser should NOT lead to additional scarring.

* * * * *

Knowing the alternative procedures available to me and with an understanding of the laser treatment protocol, I agree to participate and cooperate with Dr. _____. I have been given the opportunity to ask questions and have had them answered to my complete satisfaction. I also agree to have photographs taken, which will identify only the areas to be treated. The photographs may be used for medical records and if, in the judgment of my practitioner, medical research or education will benefit by their use, such photographs and information relating to my case may be published in professional journals or medical books or be used for any other purpose that is deemed proper in the interest of medical education, knowledge, or research, provided that I shall not be identified by name.

_____   _____

Patient signature (Printed name)   Date

_____

Witness

138 SAMPLE PATIENT INFORMATION AND CONSENT FORM FOR LASER TREATMENT OF VASCULAR LESIONS

You have a vascular lesion (hemangioma, telangiectasia, angioma, or port-wine stain), which is made up of a network of blood vessels that are close to the skin surface and therefore cause the affected skin to be pink, red, or purple in color. Many treatment methods have been tried to correct this lesion, including traditional surgery and skin grafting, injections with various substances, electrosurgery, freezing, and x-ray radiation. Unfortunately, the results have not been uniformly satisfactory using these treatments and several patients were scarred.

Lasers have been used in the treatment of vascular lesions for many years. More specific lasers utilizing a yellow light, which can selectively destroy the involved blood vessels, have been used with excellent clinical results since the early 1980s. Multiple laser treatments are usually necessary to destroy a vascular lesion. Most telangiectasias or spider veins require only one to four laser treatments, whereas port-wine stains require an average of nine to twelve treatments for significant lesional lightening. The strength of the laser power must be individualized and successive treatments over the same area several weeks or months apart may be required to select the best treatment dose for each patient. A local anesthetic to lessen the snapping sensation of the laser may be necessary in the area to be treated. Young children may require sedative medication or anesthesia.

Existing laser research and clinical evidence indicate that laser surgery is safe; however, there is no guarantee that laser treatment will resolve your condition completely. While side effects of this procedure are minimal, there is a small risk of skin texture changes or scarring, pigmentary changes (skin lightening or darkening), and infection.

* * * * *

Knowing the alternative procedures available to me and with an understanding of the laser treatment protocol, I agree to participate and cooperate with Dr. _____. I have been given the opportunity to ask questions and have had them answered to my complete satisfaction. I also agree to have photographs taken that will identify only the areas to be treated. The photographs may be used for medical records and if, in the judgment of my practitioner, medical research or education will benefit by their use, such photographs and information relating to my case may be published in professional journals or medical books or be used for any other purpose that is deemed proper in the interest of medical education, knowledge, or research, provided that I shall not be identified by name.

_____   _____

Patient signature (Printed name)   Date

_____

Witness

140 SAMPLE PATIENT INFORMATION AND CONSENT FORM FOR TATTOO TREATMENT

A tattoo is made by depositing various colored pigments under the skin surface. Many methods have been tried to remove tattoos including surgical excision, use of various acids and bleaching agents, destruction by heat or cold, overtattooing with flesh-colored pigment, sanding or dermabrading, and various lasers. The Q-switched {Nd:YAG, alexandrite, ruby} laser is the latest in a new class of state-of-the-art laser technology specifically designed for tattoo treatment. The following factors should be considered in your decision to undergo treatment.

1. It may not be possible to remove 100% of your tattoo. Certain pigments are especially "stubborn" and may require multiple treatments for particle lightening or use of an alternative laser.

2. A series of treatments may be required averaging four to six sessions for amateur tattoos and six to eight sessions for professional tattoos.

3. There may be a crust or scab on the skin requiring special care with topical antibiotic ointment, bandages, and limitation of activity in some cases for a period of 1 to 2 weeks following treatment.

4. Paradoxical darkening can occur in some facial cosmetic tattoos (eyeliner, lipliner) and, occasionally, in some colored tattoos.

5. Skin hyperpigmentation (brownish or dark discoloration) or hypopigmentation (lightening of the skin) may occur.

6. Indentation or depression of the skin may occur.

7. Skin texture change or scarring may occur.

Knowing the alternative procedures available to me and with an understanding of the laser treatment protocol, I agree to participate and cooperate with Dr. _____. I have been given the opportunity to ask questions and have had them answered to my complete satisfaction. I also agree to have photographs taken that will identify only the areas to be treated. The photographs may be used for medical records and if, in the judgment of my practitioner, medical research, education, or science will benefit by their use, such photographs and information relating to my case may be published in professional journals or medical books or be used for any other purpose that is deemed proper in the interest of medical education, knowledge, or research, provided that I shall not be identified by name.

_____   _____

Patient signature (Printed name)   Date

_____

Witness

SAMPLE PATIENT INFORMATION AND CONSENT FORM FOR LASER TREATMENT OF PIGMENTED LESIONS

You have a condition that is caused by a deposit of pigmented cells (melanocytes) at various depths under the skin surface. There have been no truly effective methods of treatment for pigmented skin conditions without significant side effects, such as scarring, prior to the development of laser technology. The following factors should be considered in your decision to undergo laser treatment.

1. Multiple treatments may be necessary (especially for pigmented birthmarks such as café-au-lait spots and nevus of Ota).

2. Treatments are separated by intervals as short as 6 to 8 weeks.

3. It may not be possible to completely remove all the pigmentation.

4. Immediately after treatment, there may be swelling and bruising, as well as crusting and scabbing, which may persist for 1 to 2 weeks.

5. Significant fading may occur for up to 6 months following treatment in some instances.

6. Possible side effects or complications of laser treatment include: (a) skin texture changes or scarring, (b) pigmentary (color) changes, including whitening or darkening of the skin (these changes are almost always temporary), (c) infection, and (d) allergy.

* * * * *

I give permission for Dr. _____ to perform laser surgery on my _____. I have been given a detailed description of the surgery and have had ample opportunity to ask questions, which have been answered to my full satisfaction. I agree to have photographs taken that will identify only the area to be treated. The photographs may be used for medical records and if, in the judgment of my physician, medical research, education, or science will benefit by their use, such photographs and information relating to my case may be published in medical journals or books or be used for any other purpose that is deemed proper in the interest of medical education, knowledge, or research. It is understood that in the event that any photographs are used for these purposes, I shall not be identified by name.

_____   _____

Patient signature (Printed name)   Date

_____

Witness

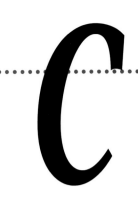

APPENDIX
LASER FORMS
AND
OPERATIVE REPORT

———

144 SAMPLE LASER TREATMENT SHEET

PATIENT _____ AGE _____ DATE _____

DIAGNOSIS _____ SURGEON _____

SKIN PIGMENT TYPE _____ SUNSCREEN ____ MAKEUP ____

AGE LESION FIRST APPEARED _____

CHANGES IN LESION _____

PREVIOUS TREATMENTS _____

ASSOCIATED MEDICAL PROBLEMS _____

CURRENT MEDICATIONS _____

ALLERGIES _____

FAMILY HISTORY _____

EXACT SIZE, COLOR, EXTENT OF LESION _____

REFERRED BY _____

RX DATE	RX AREA	PHOTO TAKEN	LASER USED	ENERGY/ POWER	SPOT SIZE	RX TIME #PULSES

SAMPLE LASER SURGERY OPERATIVE REPORT   145

PATIENT:

DATE OF OPERATION:

DIAGNOSIS:

PROCEDURE: Laser ablation of {<u>LESION</u>} on the {<u>LOCA-</u><u>TION</u>} with the {<u>TYPE</u>} laser

SURGEON:

ANESTHESIA:

OPERATIVE COURSE: After proper informed consent had been obtained, the patient was brought into the procedure room/operative suite and placed in a supine position. Protective eyewear,or eyeshields were inserted. The {<u>TYPE</u>} laser was calibrated to {<u>ENERGY/POWER</u>} at a {<u>SIZE</u>} spot size. The entire lesion on the patient's {<u>LOCATION</u>} was then treated using confluent, nonoverlapping, laser pulses. The treated area immediately appeared {<u>COLOR</u>} in color. No bleeding or char was evident.

COMPLICATIONS ENCOUNTERED: None

POSTOPERATIVE WOUND CARE:
        Bacitracin or Polysporin QID
        Petrolatum, ice packs

POSTOPERATIVE MEDICATIONS: Tylenol 650 mg po q4h
                            and qhs

DISPOSITION OF PATIENT:

RETURN APPOINTMENT: 1 week

_____   _____
Surgeon's signature   Date

146   SAMPLE SKIN LASER RESURFACING INSTRUCTION SHEET

1. Do not tan your skin prior to laser treatment or expose your skin to the sun during the first 6–8 weeks following your surgery.

2. Inform the doctor if you have EVER experienced "cold sores" around your mouth. If so, you will be prescribed a special medication, which you will be required to take during the postoperative period.

3. You will have swelling, oozing, and crusting of the treated areas of your skin for the first several days after your surgery. For this reason, many patients prefer to arrange for time off from work and other social obligations during the initial healing stages. We suggest that you arrange all your grocery and medical supply shopping PRIOR to your scheduled surgery.

4. In order to speed you recovery, we suggest that you:

   (a) Place ICE on the treated areas during the first several hours after your surgery to minimize swelling.

   (b) Keep your head elevated on an EXTRA PILLOW for the first few nights in order to further reduce swelling.

   (c) Take two TYLENOL tablets every 4 to 6 hours during the day and at bedtime for the first few days. This will help the swelling and also alleviate any discomfort you may experience. If needed, you may request a stronger prescription pain medication.

   (d) Apply a thin layer of BACITRACIN or POLYSPORIN (not Neosporin) with your fingertip or a Q-tip to the treated areas at least 2 to 4 times daily. The ointment keeps the area moist and bacteria-free, providing a better environment for wound healing.

   (e) Gently remove any crust with a clean, cool, water-soaked washcloth (no soap!) at least twice a day. This will minimize skin "tightness" and make the area feel more comfortable.

   (f) Avoid makeup on the treated areas until you return to the office for evaluation (within 1 week). At that time, you will be advised whether you can begin makeup application.

5. Please call the office IMMEDIATELY if you have any problems with the treatment or postoperative skin care.

INDEX

An Italic page number indicates an illustration.
"t" following a page number indicates a table.